I0113725

# NO MORE SUGAR COATING:

## Finding Your Happiness in a Crowded World

By Jerry Snider

THOMAS NOBLE
BOOKS

Wilmington, DE

# THOMAS NOBLE BOOKS

Copyright © 2020 Jerry Snider. All rights reserved. No portion of this book may be reproduced mechanically, electronically, or by any other means, including photocopying, without written permission from the author. It is illegal to copy this book, post it to a website, or distribute it by any other means without permission from the author.

Author Contact: AllinHealthandWellness.com

Thomas Noble Books
Wilmington, DE

ISBN: 978-1-945586-27-9

First Printing: 2020

This publication is designed to provide accurate and authoritative information regarding the subject matter covered. It is sold with the understanding that the author is not engaged in rendering professional services. If legal, accounting, medical, psychological, or any other expert assistance is required, the services of a competent professional person should be sought. Client names have been changed to protect identities.

# DEDICATION

This book is dedicated to three men who have had a profound impact on my life. I would not be who I am today without these men.

Loren Davis, my grandfather, taught me more skills and life lessons than anyone else. I continue to rely on his wisdom even 10 years after his passing.

Pete Boudreaux, my high school coach, took a young egotistical kid and helped form me into a budding man of God. While I still call him Coach, it's awesome to know that we are friends.

John Park, my first discipler, helped me mature as a follower of Christ. I miss our weekly 6-a.m. meetings but know God took you home on His time.

# TABLE OF CONTENTS

# Introduction

⏤❦⏤

*"No one ever made a difference by being like everyone else."*
*– P.T.Barnum*

Life is a funny thing. When we are young and inexperienced, we tend to think we know everything we need to know. As we age, we acquire the wisdom to know that life is not just about us, but about everyone working together for the greater good.

*No More Sugar Coating* is ultimately a book about helping you find your purpose and starting on the path to fulfilling it—a purpose that helps you, your community, and the world. Finding that purpose can be a challenge, especially if the life you have lived to this point has been focused on fitting in where society says to fit in. Sure, there are people who will tell you that they simply stumbled upon their purpose by accident; but for most of us, it is a process that takes time, energy, and confrontation of the serious reality of who we think we are versus who we know we should be.

I can think of countless people that society defines as overnight successes. Just this morning, in my daily devotional, I read *Crushing: God Turns Pressure into Power* by T.D. Jakes. Jakes talks about how he found his calling to be a pastor early in life but had to wait. He didn't want to wait, but it wasn't his time, so he practiced preaching "in the shower" or "walking through the woods." When it was his time, he was ready.

Today, he seems to be everywhere, and it appeared as if he was an overnight success. Reality is that his overnight success, like most people, took years of studying, practice, and polishing. We'll talk more about the time it takes to become the expert in your purpose in Chapter 10 – Focus is Power.

Part of living your purpose typically means going against societal norms. We've all interacted with people that have lived life without a purpose. They typically will say something like, "How did I get here?" when speaking about their life. They'd gone with the flow a little too long and now might feel it's too late to turn back.

But it's not too late. As a runner, I see this in almost every road race I compete in. People are taking back their lives and running road races for the first time ever at the age of 35, 50, or even 60. It's never too late. As the old Chinese proverb states: the best time to plant a tree is 20 years ago, but the second-best time to plant a tree is today.

Now, I've been told by many people that I have a high level of candor. You'll likely see this come out in this book. It may even cause you to think I'm a jackass. I can promise you I'm not trying to be a jackass.

I speak with a level of frankness that most people today don't like to hear. I'm not really sure where it comes from, because neither of my parents are that way. A guess would be that it comes from my late grandfather, Loren Davis (aka Papaw), whom I loved to spend time with. We lived a good 10 hours from my grandparents, but it was common for me and one of my siblings to spend eight to 10 weeks at my grandparents' house over the summer. I spent so much time with Papaw during my formative years that years later, when he was in treatment for colon cancer, his second wife Nancy made this comment about the two of us sitting side by side on the sofa: "Now, have you ever seen the same person sitting next to each other decades apart in age?"

Papaw retired as a lieutenant colonel from the Army after serving in three wars. He then had a long career as a psychology professor at Texas A&I University (now Texas A&M Kingsville). He spent his later years of military service working with civilian governments during wartime to help them re-establish a sense of normalcy in their countries. I heard many stories from him about wartime activities (sometimes the same story over and over again). One thing I learned from his military stories was that it's necessary to be upfront and tell people exactly what you need done.

My candor may have also come from his time teaching psychology. From this, he taught me about dealing with other people. How making someone else feel great about themselves will often lead them to help you in return, but you have to do so from a point of honesty. Lying to get what you want never works out in the long run, but if you help someone else feel good about themselves or help them reach their goal, they'll often jump to be at your side when you're the one in need of help.

As my wife, Jenny, says, my candor often comes off as super-opinionated. I'll tell you right now—I am well aware that a 46-year-old doesn't know all there is to know. I'd actually argue with you that I don't know much in the grand scheme of things (that's something that I realize more and more with every passing year). Heck, when I wrote my first book, *Confidence Through Health*; I had so many grammar errors in my first draft, I questioned if I even knew the English language.

However, when I do know something, I'm going to let you know that I know. Sometimes that is difficult for people to hear. It's gotten me into some unnecessary arguments when done in writing (no one else has ever had that happen over social media, right?). Proper tone can be difficult to get across in non-verbal communication. I've sent several "I'm sorry for the way that came across" emails and texts in my lifetime.

The difficulty of having a high level of candor is not just that it can hurt someone's feelings. It also makes it a challenge to be sarcastic, which is why most people that know me would not list sarcasm as one of my skills. I've sent many "that was a joke" texts and emails in my lifetime, as well. My wife, Jenny, however, is a sarcasm queen. Maybe that's why we are so great together. Opposites attract.

So where does candor leave me?

I'm not afraid to be wrong. Candor means you share honestly, but it doesn't mean you are always correct. When I engage in a conversation, I make it my responsibility to be open-minded about the topic, even when it's something I believe I'm 99 percent correct about. The key thing I try to remember is that I can always learn something from every conversation or interaction. If there is always something to be learned, it means I can't possibly know everything. It also means my perception of what is correct and the reality of what is correct could be different.

In my mind, that's the difference between having candor and being opinionated. Candor is honesty in communication, but understanding you could be wrong. Opinionated might be sharing your honest opinion, but, often, it's with a sense that you are unwilling to change that opinion.

It's also very true that someone with a lot of candor will have a difficult time getting along with someone who is opinionated, especially if that person has a need to be liked by others. It can be seen as a battle of wills, which, over time, can turn into barriers that seem to cause instant disagreements. In reality, it's often just a simple misunderstanding that has been compounded on top of previous conversations.

This book is filled with candid remarks. That's on purpose. I don't sugar coat things very well. While not everything in life is cut and dried or black and white, there are many areas of our lives today that we should treat as such. When we live in the undecided areas of life, we often fail to take advantage of the opportunity to make a positive impact on others and our world.

In my dealings with clients as a health coach and life coach, I have often seen that the biggest obstacle to a person's success is the space between their ears. What we say to ourselves, our internal beliefs, our twisting views of the past, present, and future are all ways in which we limit our abilities.

Self-limiting beliefs are often the result of not being candid with ourselves. Instead of being honest about our ability, or lack thereof, we try to validate who we are based on who we are trying to become. On paper, it sounds like this approach should work, but our minds tend to dwell on the mistakes and not the successes. This often causes us to self-sabotage our goals.

*No More Sugar Coating* is about breaking through the outer shell of ourselves and dealing with the obstacles that are holding us back. It's like that pill you don't want to take because it tastes bad, and instead of sucking it up, you put some sugar on it and wash it down. We don't want to deal with our obstacles, so we just cover them up.

It's time to stop hiding yourself.

As you read through these chapters, you'll see just some of the many ways in which we hide our true selves in order to fit in with those around us. You'll find strategies for removing the barriers you've placed between the core of who you are and the people in your life. You'll start to build the process for living an authentic life.

At the end of each chapter, there will be a simple commitment that I suggest you make. Some of these commitments may be difficult to make, or they may take a little longer to follow through on—that's okay. It's not a race with anyone else. You are living on your own timeline; my goal is to help you have a happier journey along the way.

Each commitment will have a few pieces to it: timeframe and vision. The timeframe listed gives you a parameter for implementation, while the vision guides the desired post-implementation outcome.

Commitment #1: Honesty—Make a commitment to always be truthful.

- Timeframe: Today
- Vision: What would life be like if everything you said was a truthful statement?

# CHAPTER 1

# Why Live a Life Without Sugar Coating

⚬⚬⚬

*"We cannot think of being acceptable to others until we have first proven acceptable to ourselves." – Malcolm X*

We've all seen (and probably eaten) sugar-coated foods. Whether it's candied pecans, chocolate-covered raisins, caramel popcorn, or candied apples, we all know that putting sugar on food makes it taste better. Funny thing is, most of the foods that we sugar-coat aren't especially bad tasting on their own. You can easily find pecans, raisins, popcorn, and apples in a raw, undoctored state, and they taste pretty good.

Problem is, they don't cause the immediate dopamine release in our brain that pure sugar does. It's more of a time-delayed release, like those medications that are advertised to keep working over a 24-hour period. Processed sugar gives us a quick but short-lived dopamine rush, while foods with natural sugar provide a smaller but longer-lasting dopamine release.

Our society has become hyper-focused on quick fixes. Thus, having an immediate dopamine rush to boost our spirits has become our target. For far too many people, food has taken a turn from providing nourishment to providing joy. Our health statistics show that 70 percent of Americans are overweight or obese, which puts over two-thirds of Americans at risk for chronic disease. Obesity is one of the primary causes of chronic diseases such as heart disease, hypertension, cancer, and depression.

I'm not saying that food can't be part of entertainment. It's often the case that I get misinterpreted when I talk about how food should be viewed. When I tell someone that food should be viewed as fuel/nourishment for your body, I often hear that food should be an *experience*. That every meal should be this amazing, life-altering experience. While that may be the ideal we all hope for, think back to the meals you ate over the last week. How many altered your life in a positive, earth-shattering way?

If you had dinner with a client and sealed a large sales contract, you might say that was a huge win. But was it the food experience or the people experience?

If you had that "once in a lifetime" marriage proposal dinner—you know… where the ring is hidden in the dessert?—then maybe the meal changed your life. Or was it the experience of the proposal that was life-altering?

Now, how many of those meals you ate over the last week can you identify as being detrimental to your overall health, either now (by causing some underlying immune response such as eczema) or setting the stage for future chronic disease? Did the food you ate help boost your immune system, or did it increase the inflammation in your body?

I'm not trying to scold you for what you ate. Whether you had healthy meals or not is not the point. The purpose behind this little exercise is to start showing you potential areas where societal influences may be taking hold in your life. What the statistics show is most people in the Western world are not eating a healthy diet. I know I wasn't until 2015 when God started to pull me back to His purpose for my life. The purpose that I had ignored. I'll share more about that later in the book.

When you look at what is in the food you eat, how it's prepared, and how it interacts with/affects your body, you begin to scrutinize what you eat more carefully. What is being covered up in order to give us a quick hit of joy? The more research you do into how our food is prepared, the more likely you'll stop eating those items with extra sugar coating and look for them in their natural state.

That's part of the mental shift I encourage you to make. And not just regarding food! This will apply to all areas of your life.

You may be saying to yourself, "Yeah… that's great and all, but it's *hard* to change."

Yep, change is hard. I said it. I'll say it again later, and I'll keep saying it. But part of why it's hard is that we fail to embrace the fact that change can bring about a better future. We want to hold on to the past ways of doing things because they are comfortable, but also because we know what results to expect. We know that a candied pecan will taste sweet and bring an immediate rush of "happiness." However, if you haven't eaten a raw pecan in a while, it's an unknown. "How will it taste? Will it bring me joy?"

We also fail to change what we eat because, let's face it; it's no longer normal to eat healthy. The norm, as shown by the high rates of obesity and chronic disease, is to eat what feels good in the moment. Advertising sells to us items which are typically not good for us long term, because thinking long term has become a lost art in our society. Whether it's health, finances, or even relationships, we have become a society that wants it now, without having to put in the effort for long-term gains.

In many areas of our lives, especially the working world, "What have you done for me lately?" no longer applies. It's turned into "What are you doing for me *right now*?" In regards to your health, your gut microbiome does care about what you have done for it lately, but it is also concerned with what you are doing right now. The *combined* past and present sets your whole body up for a healthy future.

When we sugar coat our food and our lives, we are basically saying we want that immediate dopamine hit of happiness to the brain. There are a few times in life that you need that immediate boost, but most of the time, you don't. You just think you do because society (keeping up with the Joneses) tells us we can't be who we really are.

There is a lot of pressure to conform to be who others say you should be or to what other people think your life should be like.

When I was in grade school, I was constantly compared to my older sister, Melissa. She was two grades ahead of me, and we often had the same teachers. Growing up, Melissa was gifted in an area I wasn't: studying.

I never learned to study and didn't really want to learn; I was having too much fun playing pick-up games of every sport you could think of with the other boys in my neighborhood (and occasionally burning old cardboard boxes with a magnifying glass).

About two months into every school year, my teacher would have a talk with me: "Why don't you study more *like your sister*?"

Looking back, I know they were not intentionally trying to put me down by comparison. But at the time, I felt I could never live up to the standard Melissa set in school for us siblings, so I dove headfirst into sports instead. I loved sports, so it was a great fit.

While it would have been very beneficial to have learned how to study at that early age, it's not who I wanted to be. I was ok with that. I knew who I wanted to be—an athlete.

That's exactly who I became, just not to the level that I'd dreamed of. I earned a scholarship to run track and cross country at Texas A&M University and had a smattering of success running in college. But when I graduated college, I was no longer an athlete. My competitive sports years were over. I was faced with getting a job and falling in line with who society said I was supposed to be. Even though God was nudging me to step out of my comfort zone and start a health and fitness business, I ignored it and did what everyone else said I should: get a job to gain some experience in the working world because, truth be told, a 2.6 GPA from college wasn't going to knock anyone's socks off.

So I fell in line with society for almost 20 years, starting at the bottom and working my way up into management positions in both corporate and non-profit organizations. But I never seemed to stay with any company for more than four or five years. My wife, Jenny, pointed that out to me once when I was struggling to see my future at one of the companies I was with. I was right around the four-year mark and she commented that she saw my frustration coming.

At the time, I blew it off as a coincidence. One company had been bought out, and I hadn't jived with the new ownership philosophy, so I left. Another one had brought in a manager from outside the organization, and we weren't getting along well, so I left. Then I found what I thought was the place I would work at until retirement. It felt like the perfect fit, until I was laid off in 2016 after three and a half years on the job.

Shortly before the layoff, I again felt God nudging me to take up the health and fitness charge for Him. I pushed back because I didn't feel ready to step out on my own. Then God did what He often does—He removed the safety net by allowing me to be laid off.

I was given a choice. Do I follow what God wants me to do, or do I find another job and be miserable living a work-life I don't really want?

In the end, I accepted God's nudge, but I did so with one very important piece in place: the will to study and become the best, most knowledgeable health and wellness professional I could be. I had to be confident and secure in myself to know that I know what I know . . . and today, I know my field really well.

That's not to say I know it all, because I don't. I spend anywhere from five to ten hours a week studying the latest health, nutrition, fitness, and wellness information available from the top doctors and researchers in the world. I also spend part of that time researching some of the non-traditional ways of achieving good health. For instance, did you know that taking a quarter-inch slice of a white potato, placing it against the sole of your foot, and covering it with a sock to hold it in place while you sleep for seven or eight hours will remove toxins from your body? It works wonders if you are starting to feel sick.

They don't teach you that in school. You learn that from being inquisitive and not accepting that society's normally prescribed way is the only way. There are many techniques to get what you want out of life. The key is not only finding what works for you but having the resolve to stand out from the crowd. When you sugar coat your life by doing what society says to do, you simply live the life society says you should have.

To not stand out may be perfectly fine with you. But I would challenge you that if you look inside yourself, you will find someone who wants more. I'm not talking about more money—that's society talking—I'm talking about the things we all want: health, freedom, and time with those we love. If you have all three of these, regardless of the amount in your bank account, I challenge you to tell me that you would not be happy.

The authors of the United States Declaration of Independence listed the three unalienable rights of all humans as "Life, Liberty, and the Pursuit of Happiness." They knew these basic goals almost 250 years ago.

Happiness may look different for each person. From the outside looking in, you might say my sister's happiness came from achievement in school (she was valedictorian of her high school class), while my happiness came from sports activities. Some athletes get to the Olympics and will comment that they are just "happy to be here," while others place their happiness on winning an Olympic medal.

When asked, most people will say they have a "happy place"; a place that brings them immense joy. I want to challenge you to begin to believe that your happy place is inside you. It's not only available when you are in a specific geographical location, but rather with you all the time.

Your happy place is who you are when you are not sugar coating your life to fit in with society. As you go through this book, I will layout the process of finding who you are without the sugar coating. All you need to do is commit to coming out the other side as a happy person.

Pretty simple request, really. Who wouldn't want to be a happy person? Well, the scary thing is most people in our Western world today are not living a genuinely happy life. Many are simply trying to get by and survive. Getting by and surviving are not typically phrases that are linked to happiness.

A common misconception about achieving happiness is that if I'm happy, someone else can't be happy, because my happiness must come at someone else's expense. This does not have to be a true statement. Sure, it can be true at times. In a sporting event, it's not always realistic to believe that the winner and loser are both happy with the result. But when you look at health, freedom, and spending time with loved ones, we can all achieve happiness without hurting anyone else.

In Matthew, chapter 22, of the Bible, there is a scene where an expert in religious law was questioning Jesus:

> *"Teacher, which is the greatest commandment in the Law?"*
>
> *Jesus replied: "'Love the Lord your God with all your heart and with all your soul and with all your mind.' This is the first and greatest commandment. And the second is like it: 'Love your neighbor as yourself.' All the Law and the Prophets hang on these two commandments." (Matt 22: 36-40 NIV)*

"Love your neighbor as yourself" is a very important piece of the happiness puzzle. First, it indicates that you love yourself for who you are. In order to truly love yourself, you must first know who you are at the core. After you love yourself, you need to love your neighbor for who they are. The genuine version of your neighbor.

If you go through life loving your neighbor as yourself and are doing so without sugar-coating your life, you will not achieve happiness at your neighbor's expense. In fact, the more likely result would be creating happiness in both your life and their life.

We all know what a sugar-coated life looks like. One quick glance through any social media platform will turn up multiple examples. You'll find people posting only the highlight reels of their lives to make it appear like they have everything one could possibly desire: a perfect family life, a perfect job, perfect meals, etc. The problem with perfect is that no one has a perfect life. We all have ups and downs. It's rare, however, for someone to showcase the downs of their life.

We even see sugar-coated lives in the people we run into at the grocery store. Those friends we haven't seen in a few weeks ask us how life is going, and we reply, "it's going well," when a lot of the times, it's not really going well. We could be in the middle of a crisis, but societal norms prevent us from being that open in a grocery store environment. So, instead, we sugar coat our response, potentially leading our friend to wonder why their life can't be as good as ours . . . when ours is crumbling.

I went through this experience at church a few years ago. My friend, Tom, called me out instead of letting the conversation simply go by like every other short interaction. As we shook hands, he asked how I was doing. I replied with a simple, "Oh, I'm doing ok." Instead of letting go of my hand and moving on down the hallway, he held firm and looked me in the eye. He then asked, "Are you really doing ok?" In the next split second, I thought of two answers: "Yes, I'm ok," or the truth: "Well . . . things have been pretty tough lately."

I went with the truth and not just because I didn't want to lie in church. I knew he was genuine in his inquiry, and I should be genuine in my reply. He cared, and I should honor that with the truth. It only took a few extra minutes of conversation for Tom to get the gist of what was going on in my life, and he promised to pray for me over the next few days.

The following Sunday, I saw Tom again as I was entering the church sanctuary. We shook hands, and, as we looked each other in the eye, the question came: "How are you doing?" Once again, I was honest in my reply: "I'm doing good. Not great, but I'm doing good." Tom released my hand and nodded with a smile. Ever since then, we greet each other with that same question and hold each other accountable to an honest answer. The funny thing is, I have no recollection of what negative issue was going on in my life at that time, but I do remember the impact that Tom made on my life by simply breaking through the sugar-coat.

It seems simple because it is. However, it's not always easy to share your core feelings and emotions with others. I'm not saying you need to share your most intimate details and struggles with any stranger you come in contact with. There is a level of sharing that we all know is okay given the type of relationship you have with the other individual. I'm simply acknowledging the need for honesty both with others and with ourselves. A life without sugar coating is an honest life.

You might be thinking you would love to be so honest, but you have strong opinions and views that could easily disrupt the relationships you have. In order to "keep the peace" with friends and family, you have been sugar coating your opinions for years.

My first response to that is that I'm glad you have opinions. But remember that opinions are built from your current perspective on life with input from past experiences. Your opinions could be wrong,

I'm not saying they *are* wrong, they just could be. Keep that in mind when you start removing the sugar coating.

Secondly, having opinions but never sharing them doesn't help anyone. It's like being the kid in class who has a question but never raises his hand. He never gets clarification on his question, which leads him to answer incorrectly on the next test. The key is sharing your opinion without purposefully seeking to offend others. Your opinion, presented in the right way, even has the power to prevent your loved ones from doing something detrimental.

As with most families, my extended family has its share of health problems scattered throughout. I often offer to provide guidance where I can, but sometimes it comes off as harsh. At times, the family member wants help, but either isn't ready for the truth or isn't used to hearing straightforward responses. You can't let that scare you when you know your opinions could help the situation improve.

If you are sharing opinions from an honest and open heart that is free of sugar coating, you will be less likely to offend the recipient. They may not like your opinion, but they'll respect you for sharing it. The byproduct of that interaction is the breaking down of another layer of the sugar coating of both of your lives. If you want to love yourself and others well, break down the layers of sugar coating.

Commitment #2: Stop judging yourself

- Timeframe: Today
- Vision: Imagine your future self being happy with who you are

## CHAPTER 2

# What Story is Your Life Telling?

*"Tension is who you think you should be.*
*Relaxation is who you are" – Chinese proverb*

The story of your life is likely different from the story your life is telling. One refers to an obituary-type detailing of things you did in your lifetime. The other depicts who you are and what your purpose is. If you don't know your purpose, it's highly likely no one else does either.

The story of your life is the past. It's the lines on your resume. It's medals on your wall or the pictures from vacation travels. These are great, fun accomplishments and experiences that can have a shaping effect on who you become. These are also things that can be hidden, preventing your true core-person from being seen. You are not just the sum of all your accomplishments.

The story your life is telling can be a far more complex story than simply a listing of things you've done. Who are you? What are you working towards? What do you believe? Do you stand for something that others can easily see?

The answers to these questions will begin to shape the story you want to be told if you allow people to see those answers in action.

If you let them, your experiences throughout life will influence the story you are telling. God has taught me over the years that life is about sharing our experiences with others. I've made some big and small incorrect decisions in my life that weren't necessarily bad decisions, just not the correct ones for my life. But I believe if my life experiences can prevent a pitfall in your life, then there is a reason for this book.

One of the questions all adults have asked a child is, "What do you want to be when you grow up?" This is an innocent question which receives a variety of answers depending on the age of the child. From toddler to elementary school age, you will likely receive one of these answers: cowboy, fireman, ninja, dancer, football player, fashion designer, movie star, artist, etc. As children get older, the answers for some change to professions with which they have had a personal connection or passion. For instance, a child who grows up near a farm develops a special love for animals and might decide to become a veterinarian. Or a child who loves to build structures with Legos might become an engineer or architect.

For me, there was never that dream-profession, except, of course, becoming a professional athlete. In my early years, the dream was to be a professional soccer player, a dream that six months in Scotland as an 11-year-old helped to build. Then I discovered my ability to run and competed in eighth-grade track in 1988. I was successful fairly quickly, and then later that year, after watching the Olympics, the dream switched to Olympic athlete.

I was a bit naive, of course, but I thought I had a great chance of making it because I had three sports that I loved–soccer, track, and waterskiing. I figured, for sure, I would make it in one of them. The soccer team I played on, the Baton Rouge Blue, had just won the 1988 state championship, and we traveled to Florida to play in the U.S. Southern Regional Tournament. That same summer, I attended a waterski school for a week as my eighth-grade graduation present. As my skills progressed quickly that week, I envisioned how great I would be if only given the opportunity to ski on a regular basis. Then there was running. I had only lost one distance race in eighth grade and thought that, with more training, I would easily improve quickly.

You've obviously figured out that I didn't make the Olympics in any of these sports, or I would have led with that as part of my introduction for the book. But that is okay. Some dreams will become reality, and some dreams are just that… dreams.

Then there is the reality that most people in America live, the reality they never dreamt of. Most aren't too happy about their reality compared to their dreams from childhood. Some of the realities of adulthood can be downright depressing: bills, jobs, planning for retirement, etc. That's why we don't tell children about them, but rather have them focus on their dreams.

I recall a situation once where an employee I managed asked about the likelihood of getting promoted from a part-time employee to full-time status. In giving her reasoning for why she deserved the position, she mentioned her reality of being a recent college graduate. Her monthly student loan payments had begun, and she needed more income to meet her new responsibilities. She said the phrase we have likely all said at some point: "It's no fun being an adult."

Her reality had changed. She was forced to act due to her commitment to repay the loan she took out to pay for her college tuition. That same college degree she graduated with, and owed money for, did not provide a position that gave her the financial ability to pay back the loan. This is just one example of the catch-22 scenario so many Americans find themselves in.

So, how can we make our reality something we have dreamt about? My hope is that I can help you answer that question, but, in doing so, you will have to make a commitment as well.

You have to commit to not being normal. You need to be weird.

Why? Because that's what it takes to reach your dreams. Think about my dream of being an Olympic Athlete. Statistically, a very small percentage of people on this Earth become Olympic Athletes. Just 14,000 athletes out of the 7.5 billion on the planet participated in the 2016 Summer and 2018 Winter Olympic Games. That's about one out of every 535,000 people alive at the time. That's pretty weird, although most people would say it's more unique to be an Olympic athlete than it is to be weird.

Are you willing to do something so different that you are the only one of 535,000 other people doing it? You are already unique in some way. There are not two people alive that are exactly the same in every detail. The difference is those people who aren't afraid of being weird have already broken that sugar coating off of their lives. They are not afraid to show who they are at every moment of every day.

That's the commitment level this book is about. Making the commitment to be weird, to showcase who you are, to use your gifts and talents to help the community around you, and to reach your insanely crazy dreams other people make fun of.

Think about it for a minute. If being weird meant that you could not only live the dreams of your childhood but also live the life you currently dream of… would you do it? I know it probably means some hard work and facing potential ridicule from others, but wouldn't your dream, YOUR DREAM, be worth being a little weird??

My guess is you said yes. The benefit of living your dream life far outweighs dealing with a little ridicule. So how do we get you there?

Like many who are living a life they didn't dream of, there is often a feeling that you have no control. Oddly enough, that's ok. There is a misconception that the people who are reaching for their dreams have everything under control. The reality is that successful people know what aspects of their lives they do have control over. They "stay in their lane" so to speak by having total control of just those areas of life. Then they worry very little, if at all, about the areas they can't control.

The milk spilled. No sense in crying about it. Clean it up and move on with life.

You need to gain control of your life by coming to an understanding that people rarely think or even worry about your life. Sure, your immediate family (spouse, kids, parents) will think about you at times throughout the day. But other than that, very few people actually waste any time with thoughts of you except during those moments when you are directly relevant to the task they are managing.

If you understand that they are not worrying about you, then why are you worrying about them? I still catch myself occasionally thinking, "I wonder what that person thinks of me" after a meeting. In reality, they either aren't thinking about me, or they are asking themselves the same exact question in reverse—trying to figure out what I think about them. The whole time, we tell ourselves we are caring about other people, but really, we are just concerned about how we are portrayed in their minds.

People who are successful, secure, and know what story they want to tell through their lives will tell you straight up what they think of you. They'll let you know if you have a place on their team (as I'll discuss in Chapter 8: Who is on Your Team?). They move on towards their goal without spending unnecessary time dwelling on the past pieces of their story. They show the world who they are, what they believe, and share what their goals/dreams are. Then they execute towards those goals and dreams.

People who are successful at telling their story through their life know what's important to them. They also know what's not important to them; that way they do not get sucked up into things that, while maybe valid issues, are not going to help tell their story or reach their goals.

The first step in trying to decide if something is important is to define what that something is. If you say your faith is important to you, then you need to have a definition for what faith means to you. One definition of faith is "complete trust or confidence in someone or something." By this definition, if you have faith in something, you should be confident. So why are so many people in our world lacking confidence? I contend it is for two reasons. Many have their faith placed in the wrong things, while others have never defined what their faith means to them.

Placing your faith in the wrong thing is something that is done every day by almost everyone. We put our faith in almost every decision we make, from which pen to use to write with, to letting someone else drive us to our next meeting. When you only take one pen into a meeting, and the ink dries up, what do you do? It's a pretty simple and easy issue, but it doesn't change that you put your faith in that one pen making it all the way through that meeting.

Alternatively, if your faith is in God, does your life tell that story? Not just your spiritual life, but your life as a whole?

For many of us in a politically correct society, it is difficult to wear your faith on your sleeve. Our politically correct culture tells us it's not okay to offend others, which creates a fine line between showing your convictions and sugar-coating who you are to fit into the world's expectations.

I'm not suggesting we should look for ways to offend other people. Just the opposite is true if you are secure in what story your life is telling. You won't be offended by anyone else because you understand that they have convictions just as you do. The offense typically occurs when one of two things are in place:

- the receiving person in the conversation is not secure in their beliefs and therefore gets offended because they feel threatened
- the giving person in the conversation can tell that the receiving person has a sugar-coated life and therefore is "faking" the conversation

One way to know if you are strong in your convictions is to ask your friends, both close and casual, if they know what you stand for. Can they tell you what you believe to be true? Can they tell you what you care about?

In order to have this conversation you have to be ready for both constructive criticism and negative feedback. You might hear something you don't feel is a true representation of who you think you are. It's also possible you may get a macro-level answer (high-level view) when you are looking for some micro-input (the nitty gritty of who you are). On the other hand, it's a good sign if they peg one of your core beliefs.

The concept of macro versus micro is commonly applied to many areas of our lives. Looking at economics and nutrition, which can both be tricky subjects, there always seems to be a debate over which is more important—a focus on macro or on micro. There are a lot of parallels between economics, nutrition, and how each of us is perceived.

It's important to know the effect that a macro-life has on how your story is being told. Not that a macro-life is bad, but when the macro and micro do not align well, neither do your economics, nutrition, nor the story your life is telling.

You've likely heard someone say, "I can't eat carbs. They just aren't good for me." This is a macro approach that doesn't take the micro needs into consideration. The human body actually runs on carbs. The issue is that some carbs are much better than other carbs. And yes, there are carbs that should never be allowed in your body.

Focusing on the macros of nutrition is an attempt to be healthy by looking at the big picture of food—protein, fat, carbohydrates, fiber. The idea is to take some of the details out of the picture by making it simple. In an ideal world, you create a healthy body by sticking to eating certain percentages of protein, fat, carbs, and fiber.

In economics, that thinking is shown by looking at the indicators of the overall economy. At the national level, financial success or growth is shown by the stock market numbers, housing market numbers, unemployment numbers, and gross domestic product. If most or all of these numbers are trending in a positive direction, we see a booming economy.

Digging into what makes up a fat, we find all kinds of substances. Some of these have nutritional value and some don't. In fact, some are non-nutritious to the point of causing damage. There are saturated fats, unsaturated fats, poly-unsaturated fats, and so on. Fat can come from different food sources—animals, plants, nuts. It's quite possible to limit your meals to 15 percent fat content while thinking you'll be getting 100 percent nutrition from that fat, but actually get zero percent, because you are eating the wrong kinds of fats. Now you are creating a micronutrient issue.

Following a meal plan focused on micro-nutrition makes you look at the basic vitamins, minerals, enzymes, etc. in the food you eat. Are you getting enough Vitamin A, Calcium, and Omega 3 to have properly functioning cells. Whereas macro-nutrition is looking at the body as a whole, micro-nutrition is watching the success or failure of each individual cell?

To go back to economics, while macroeconomics is looking at the country as a whole, microeconomics would be looking at your individual financial situation. Every economist would agree the country would be doing extremely well financially, if every single individual (or household) was thriving financially. That's not the case though; we all know someone (maybe ourselves) that is burdened with debt, living paycheck to paycheck.

When enough of these struggling people are in close proximity to each other, there becomes an economic crisis in that region. The crisis could be caused by a number of marco issues—stock of a particular company drops, which causes job-loss and creates a housing issue; or, maybe a poorly run local government.

A stock typically rises and falls in value based on the perception of success of the company—how it looks from the outside. That is, until a fault comes to light that was being hidden. It may or may not have been hidden on purpose by those in charge of the company, but something happens to devalue the appearance of the company, and the stock plummets. Usually, these faults fall into one of three areas: poor planning, greed, or a scandal. You could even argue that most scandals arise from poor planning and greed combined.

You may appear to look great on the outside, but what's going on inside? Poor planning and greed sound a lot like the reasons most people are shown to be in bad physical health. Not living on a proper meal plan and, therefore, succumbing to greed (or desires of the taste buds) when eating. When a cell does not get proper nutrition for an extended period of time, it becomes inflamed, deformed/damaged, or dies. If enough of these cells are in close proximity to each other, we see the formation of chronic disease. It's very similar to the economic crisis that can happen in a particular region.

While one financially destitute household in a neighborhood will not likely cause any changes for their neighbors, multiple struggling households in that neighborhood will cause an economic crisis. While one inflamed/damaged cell of an organ will not likely cause health problems, multiple inefficient cells cause the organ to begin failing.

Writer and philosopher, George Santayana, stated, "Those who cannot remember the past are condemned to repeat it." The history of economics shows us that there are multiple ways to revive a financially struggling region. Some work long term and some don't. What has not seemed to work well is simply providing those struggling families a temporary relief package, such as a stimulus or tax break. The steps that work to bring a neighborhood back to vibrance are the teaching of financial literacy, job skills, entrepreneurship, and small business support.

When it comes to your health, medication is supposed to be the temporary relief package. All medications for chronic diseases are meant to be used for a short term, and not the remainder of your life. The steps that do work to bring back good health are learning how to eat properly, exercising regularly, maintaining a healthy weight, and stress management.

Unfortunately, we have too many people with a mindset of "The government will fix my financial life" or "Medication will fix my health". The reality is, each person is capable of fixing their financial situation because of free enterprise. Each person can also improve their health situation simply by controlling what is consumed and engaging in regular exercise.

Both your health and your finances are a direct reflection of where you place your focus and discipline. If you focus on the macros, you may appear to be doing well. It's when you understand and are disciplined about applying the principles of the micros that you will experience long-term success.

Are your life's macro story and micro storytelling on the same storyline? Success is possible if they are both aligned with your core values. If that is the case, you are more than likely living a life without any sugar coating. If your macro story is different from your micro- story, you are likely struggling to figure out what your life is all about, how to find success, and/or who is on your side.

One of the issues I see with living for a macro life is that it often pushes you to keep up with the Joneses. In today's society, the Joneses tend to be famous actors and athletes. Why do they get all the endorsement deals? Because most people today desire to have what they have, the impression becomes that if you have the material possessions a famous person has, your life will be better.

I love this quote from Jim Carrey: "I think everybody should get rich and famous and do everything they ever dreamed of so they can see that it's not the answer." Here's one of the most famous people in Hollywood telling us a macro life is not the answer.

On the day in the future on which you pass away, will the people who are left behind know the story of your life as you would want it to be told? Or will they simply know the different things you accomplished?

Commitment #3: Share an opinion derived from one of your core beliefs with a friend. Pick something which that friend doesn't already know about you.

- Timeframe: In the next 48 hours
- Vision: Sharing freely with friends when times are both great and difficult

# CHAPTER 3

# Living a Selfless Life

*"Do I not destroy my enemies when I make them my friends?"*
*– Abraham Lincoln*

September 24, 2013.

That's one of those dates I'll never forget. It likely doesn't mean anything to you. For me, that's the day I suffered my second spontaneous pneumothorax (collapsed lung).

It was just over two years since my first spontaneous pneumothorax. Both times, it happened during my sleep. It just so happened that my wife, Jenny, was out of town visiting family. I drove myself to the hospital, where a doctor friend of mine was able to get me through triage quickly and into a room. Another doctor came in and inserted a chest tube to re-inflate my lung so that I could rest comfortably before surgery later that afternoon.

As Jenny was hysterically driving back to town as quickly as she could, my pastor, Grant, came to visit me. Looking back, though I knew I wasn't going to die during that episode, I was very concerned, and shared that with my pastor that morning. I was also very worried that Jenny would get in an accident due to driving under such emotional stress. Well, Jenny made it safely, just in time for the surgery; and soon after, my surgeon performed what's called a pleurodesis. In layman's terms, he glued my lung to my rib cage so that if it popped again, it wouldn't collapse.

A few days later, Grant came to visit again. He inquired about my emotional state, fearing death, and how he could pray for me. I told him not to pray for me, but to pray for the person in the next room. I had noticed they had so many visitors that they spilled into the hallway, and they all carried an especially sad demeanor, indicating a very serious diagnosis. I knew in my heart I would be ok but didn't know what was going on with that other patient.

Grant then walked over to the dry-erase board that nurses use to keep daily notes. He wrote down Phil 2:3-4. He told me what those verses read.

> *"Do nothing out of selfish ambition or vain conceit.*
> *Rather, in humility value others above yourselves,*
> *not looking to your own interests but each of you*
> *to the interests of the others."*
> *Philippians 2:3-4*

Then, he said I was living those verses by my actions. In one of my deepest moments of need, I was more concerned about the patient in the room next to me. I didn't know these verses by heart at the time, but I do now. I've tried to live these verses since that day, but I still struggle with it even though I purposefully think about this verse daily. If I struggle with it, then I know people who are not intentionally trying to live this verse are definitely struggling with it.

I recall a trip to visit Jenny's family. We traveled down on Saturday just to turn back around on Sunday to come home. It was a pretty quick turnaround for a four-hour drive each way, but it was a necessary trip to visit a sick relative. You might say that making the trip was a way of living out this verse.

Well, a lack of this verse came into play on Sunday morning. On the drive home, Jenny informed me that I was completely self-absorbed, which was the 100-percent opposite of the life I had been trying to lead. What upset me the most was this was my wife calling me selfish, the one person who knew me better than anyone. I couldn't let it roll off my back.

I sat back and really evaluated my motives. Was I just putting on a show for others? Had I been faking my faith for years? Was I really living a Christian life?

A big part of why she called me self-absorbed was because I went on a long run that morning before we headed home. Her parents live in a much hillier part of the state than we do, referred to as The Texas Hill Country.

Sundays are typically my long run day, so I wanted to take advantage of the opportunity to run a long run up and down the hills. The day before, she jokingly asked if I was running for two hours, to which I told her I had no intention of doing so. The plan was to run between 12 and 14 miles, depending on how my legs felt, likely taking around an hour and a half.

That morning, the weather was overcast. For safety's sake, I didn't get moving as early as I would have liked. But when I did finally run, my legs felt great. I even experienced a few moments where I fell asleep running. I got into such a rhythm that my mind lost track of time.

After about seven miles, I really felt great and decided to turn around at eight miles and do the whole loop through the hills again.

It gave me a total run of 16 miles. I was keeping an eye on my watch and the time of day towards the end so that I could finish with enough time to get on the road home when Jenny wanted to. I finished the 16-mile run in an hour and 53 minutes.

Upon entering the house, I found everyone eating breakfast. Now, I've run there many times on a Sunday morning and often do not get back in time for breakfast. Jenny also knows I do not like to eat right after finishing a run; I need a little bit of time to cool off.

After I cooled off, showered, and ate breakfast, we got on the road back home. That's when the conversation happened.

I don't tell this story to have you pick sides between me and my wife. It's not about who was right and who was wrong. It's about selfish behavior and communication with others. You see, in my mind, I had to accomplish two things for Jenny on that Sunday morning: run less than two hours, and leave at the time she wanted. Both of those were accomplished, so I didn't see how I was being self-absorbed.

What Jenny saw was that I ran for two hours (only long-distance runners would calculate an hour and 53 minutes as not being two hours), and I missed breakfast with the family. While breakfast with the family was not one of the requested tasks for me to get done, it was a short trip, and the unspoken request of spending time with her family was something she expected of me.

Turns out we were both being selfish—go figure. I had indeed been selfish to attempt to run longer than she'd expected without communicating that to her. We often communicate by phone when I'm running, so the fact I was already running when I decided to extend the run is no excuse. Was I selfish when I missed breakfast, even having missed it during several trips in the past? Yes. Just because I had done it before; didn't make it unselfish this time.

Was she selfish in wanting me to run shorter so that there was no rush in leaving? Yes, but since she is not a long-distance runner, she often doesn't understand some of the "crazy running things" I do. Was she selfish in wanting me to help get the kids ready instead of being on my run? You could easily say yes, especially since she was in an emotional state, given that her family member was in the hospital.

Selfish behavior is at the core of who we are, but we were not made that way. According to Genesis 1:26-27, God made man in His image and likeness. If God made us to be selfish, then it would stand to reason that He is inherently selfish.

Does God think of himself first before thinking of us? That's what it would mean for Him to be selfish. There are far too many examples where God shows that He is not selfish. The fact that He created mankind to live on the Earth and enjoy His creation should be example enough that He is not selfish. But when Adam and Eve ate from the Tree of Knowledge, it plunged mankind into a world of sin. With sin in the world, it may seem as if God is selfish at times.

Don't get confused between selfish and just. God is a just God in the same way that parents provide justice when disciplining their children. Proverbs 22:6 reads, "Train up a child in the way he should go, even when he is old he will not depart from it." Without getting into a debate on child-rearing, we've all seen teens act in ways that make us think, "That's just how they were raised." That statement in your mind is proof that, to some extent, we are a product of our environment. The apple doesn't fall far from the tree, right? We were not created to be selfish, but our sinful environment has corrupted our behavior.

Another example of God's selflessness is Jesus Christ. Jesus walked the Earth to show us the way. Christians who have accepted Jesus as their personal savior know that Jesus is the way to Heaven. I believe he came to Earth to show us another way as well—the way to live while we are here on Earth.

When Jesus shared the Lord's Prayer with his disciples (Matt 6:10), he used the phrase "on earth as it is in heaven." Jesus' ministry was about showing us how to operate here on Earth. He tried to show us that not only will we not have to deal with earthly issues in Heaven, we don't have to deal with them on Earth if we have enough faith in God.

When we are selfish, we put our faith in ourselves. Our own abilities become the focus of our decisions, successes, and confidence. On the other hand, when our faith is in God, we truly exist to help others. That's the way Jesus lived. He had 100 percent faith in God, and it never wavered.

A common question I hear from non-Christians is, "Why did God allow Jesus, His own Son, to be crucified?" It is a hard question to understand, because our selfish nature would never allow our own child to be killed, especially if we had the power to save them. What you must remember is that God is selfless. Had He reached down and saved Jesus from dying on the cross, it would have been the ultimate "I'm going to take my ball and go home" move.

I know that analogy may not reach everyone. For anyone who grew up playing neighborhood ball of any sort, the thought of being in the middle of the game, and the kid with the ball gets so upset with the game that he grabs his ball and goes home, is devastating. It'd be the most selfish thing he could do at that moment.

Just as the ball is a crucial part of the game, Jesus is the crucial part of getting to Heaven. Without Jesus' death on the cross and resurrection to Heaven, we would have no pathway to Heaven. Does this mean that once someone accepts Jesus as their Savior, they can now take Jesus and go home as if he was their ball?

Not at all. As believers in Christ, we are called on to love others as we love ourselves (Matt 22:39). Pretty hard to be selfish if you are loving someone else the way you love yourself. It's actually downright impossible. That's the thing about faith in God—He makes the impossible possible.

When the Bible states to lay down your life for another (John 15:13), do you think it might be metaphorical and not literal? When was the last time you put someone else's problems ahead of your own?

It's easy to do if you have kids, especially for moms. I deal with a lot of moms who have cared for everyone else in their family but disregarded their own health and wellness in the process. That's not the best scenario and is actually cautioned against in the Bible, as well. Failing to care for ourselves and only looking to care for others is not healthy either.

Jesus said, if you don't take care of your own house first, you are worse than an unbeliever. This sounds selfish, but trying to help others without being in proper health—physically, emotionally, and/or spiritually—is never going to be fully successful. You have to be greedy about caring for yourself. This doesn't mean being selfish. There is a fine line between the two. Self-care is understanding the needs that you have, and reaching your goals in a healthy way is the only way that you will be successful in helping others reach their goals.

On the other hand, reaching your goals in a selfish way can hurt others along the way. This almost always alienates you from the people around you, which in turn denies you love for yourself.

This all begs the question: How do you live a truly selfless life? It actually starts by loving yourself.

You can't love someone else if you don't first love yourself. Getting emotionally tied up in someone else's life to the point you ignore your own life is a quick way to find yourself depressed and alone. Members of my extended family have dealt with severe depression at times. Sure, we all get depressed from time to time—that's called situational depression. But severe depression is a long-term, deeper issue. While depression can start from many different circumstances, it puts you in a place of despair and despondency. The emotional state you enter into can easily make it feel as if you are not worth anything, and that makes it hard to love yourself.

If you are supposed to love others as you love yourself, but you don't actually love yourself, how exactly are you going to love others?

The answer is, you're not—at least not very well. You might be able to fake it for a little bit, but it eventually becomes difficult.

So what do you do? You can tell yourself you are living Phil 2:3-4 to the letter because you value everyone else more than yourself, but the true meaning of the verse is not that you should lower the value you see in yourself in order to, by default, raise others' value. Instead, you must raise the value of others above the current value you put on your own self, then, as you continue to increase your own value, simply do the same for the value you see in others.

We start by loving ourselves well. Then we love others the same way.

We must take an active role in caring for the issues and situations that others find themselves in. Does this mean we must "fix" every situation for every person we know or come in contact with? No. It means coming alongside them and loving them through the situation. Each of us has different gifts which we can use to help people through situations, but they won't work for everyone.

One of my gifts is to help people transform their health and wellness. While there are a lot of people in this world that need help with their health, I'm not gifted enough to work with everyone. And that's ok. The key for me is being open to work with everyone and letting God place the correct people in the correct place.

In the business world, it's known as working with your ideal client. While I may have the knowledge to work with everyone with regards to improving their health, not everyone is a good fit for me. Does that mean I de-value the people who don't work with me? Just the opposite. I often value potential clients so much that I refer them to other health and fitness professionals that will be able to do a better job at providing what the clients are looking for.

For example, with my knowledge, I can easily put together a training program for someone who wants to become a bodybuilder. But, it's not what I'm best at, and I know other people who are far better at it than I. When I refer that potential client to someone who better suits them, we all win. Sure, I might lose out on some money from not having them as a client, but would I have shown them value by not making them the best that they could be?

Loving others well can only happen if you are loving yourself well. In order to love yourself well, you must break down the barriers that you have created.

What barriers, do you ask? Those beliefs we have inside our mind that keep us in our comfort zone. Sure, it's great to be comfortable. I like the comfort of knowing exactly what will happen next in my life, although it rarely happens exactly the way I visualize it. I might get the end result, but I often go on a slightly, or drastically, different path than I'd first imagined.

Moving outside of our comfort zones means shedding that exterior coating that we've created and use to define ourselves.

Think back to when you were a child. If you were anything like me or my children, you changed identities almost as often as you moved between rooms. First, I was Batman, then a cowboy, then a professional athlete. Often, all in the same hour.

Now, I'm Jerry. I'm a husband and father. I'm a Christian. I'm "the health guy." I'm an athlete. I'm an author. I'm a business owner. There are a lot of labels for who I am. Those are all descriptive traits, though. Who I really am is who I believe I am in my mind at any given moment.

Sometimes, that's a "lazy bum." At times, it's "the most knowledgeable person no one listens to." Other times, it's a "horrible father" or "horrible husband." And then other times, it's a "complete and total failure."

These self-limiting beliefs could take over my life if I let them. But instead, I treat them as what they are: an obstacle that is preventing me from lifting up someone else.

Commitment #4: Volunteer at an organization that fits with your values

- Timeframe: In the next 7 days
- Vision: Make a long term decision to volunteer on a regular basis

# CHAPTER 4

# Self-Limiting Beliefs

❦

*"A man is but the product of his thoughts.*
*What he thinks, he becomes." – Mahatma Gandhi*

Back in the early- to mid-1900s, it was argued that no man could ever run fast enough to break the four-minute mile. Then, Sir Roger Bannister did it in 1954. Since then, over 1,500 men have broken the four-minute mark, and the age range for these men is 16 to 41 years old. Granted, that's a small percentage of total humans to ever inhabit Earth… It still continues to be possible.

For decades, people have been trying to travel around Earth. The human mind has a fascination with seeing how far or fast the body can go. Although it was attempted several times, the first non-stop hot air balloon trip around Earth didn't happen until 1999. Pilots Brian Jones and Bertrand Piccard flew the Breitling Orbiter 3 balloon safely around the world in just over 19 days. Then, in 2002, in The Spirit of Freedom balloon, Steve Fossett became the first solo pilot to accomplish the feat.

Then there is the story of Roderick Sewell. You've likely never heard of Sewell unless you follow the triathlon community. Sewell was born missing bones in both legs, a condition which led to a double amputation at an early age. On October 13, 2019, the 27-year-old Sewell completed the Ironman Triathlon World Championships in Kona, Hawaii. This race includes a 2.4-mile swim in the ocean, a 112-mile bike course through some of Hawaii's most treacherous landscapes, and a 26.2-mile run. For the bike course, Sewell used a handbike, and he ran with the help of his running blades. Could you imagine being a double amputee—above the knee—and completing a race with three different elements over the course of 140.6 miles?

"You'd be amazed how many people ask me if I need help," Sewell said. "Sometimes, people need help, but I'm doing Kona. It's all about how you see yourself. If I see myself as disabled, I might need help. But if I see myself like the rest of these guys out there competing, who knows what you'll be capable of."

(https://www.runnersworld.com/runners-stories/a29388043/roderick-sewell-kona-chmapionships/)

Bannister broke the impossible four-minute mile barrier. Jones, Piccard, and Fossett circumnavigated Earth without the help of engine power. Sewell completed the Ironman World Championships as a double amputee.

These examples show us that anything is possible, IF you allow your mind to think past the barriers in your life. That's a key ingredient in your health: barriers. What barriers were you taught as a child? What barriers have you learned from friends? What barriers have you created on your own?

Barriers are meant to be limiting.

A bowling alley has gutters as barriers next to each lane so that the bowling ball doesn't go into your neighbor's lane. This limits your ball from interfering with someone else's game.

An IndyCar race track has a concrete and metal fence barrier around it to limit the amount of debris from a car wreck entering stands filled with spectators.

An elementary school has locked doors to serve as barriers so that no one can enter the school without getting permission from office staff.

Someone might use sunscreen as a barrier to prevent sunburn or exposure to potential skin cancer when they are at the beach.

Barriers are limiting. This is especially true of the barriers we create in our mind. You might also call them self-limiting beliefs. The term self-limiting belief is popular in the coaching and counseling worlds. You may or may not have heard of this idea before. It refers to our ability to have thoughts or beliefs that limit us. We all do this. Sometimes in big ways and sometimes in small ways. Here's a few examples of thoughts you might think that are self-limiting:

"It's going to be a tough day."
"I can't speak in front of a crowd."
"I'm not good at…"
"I'm a failure."
"I'm not good enough to achieve my dreams."

Self-limiting beliefs are negative. They close you off to your potential, not only limiting you, but also preventing those around you from being lifted up as well. Where do these thoughts come from? Are these types of thoughts Godly thoughts?

If you believe that God is omniscient (all knowing), then it would be difficult to imagine God struggling with self-limiting thoughts. If He knows everything, it would be hard for Him to limit Himself in His thoughts. It's like trying to convince yourself that 2 + 2 = 6.

Once you know something as a fact (that truly *is* a fact), you won't be convinced otherwise.

If humans were created by God, even made in the image of God, why do we struggle so much with self-limiting thoughts? For that answer you must understand the fall of man—the lives of Adam and Eve in the Garden of Eden. By eating the apple from the Tree of Knowledge, Adam and Eve didn't just learn about their naked condition. They didn't simply allow sin to come into the world either. There was also a change in our human form that made us imperfect and no longer a mirror image of God.

Does being made in the image of God mean that we are made to die? Just the opposite. Adam and Eve were made to live forever, perfect bodies without flaws that were created with healing power from within. That might be impossible to imagine. The intricacies of the human cell, not to mention all the bodily systems, leads me to believe that we have a healing power within our bodies that is far too often limited by our inability to believe healing is possible.

This begs the question: did the human body change as a result of the eating of the apple from the Tree of Knowledge just as the human mind did?

Let's look at what we have proven through science as of today. We know that the human digestive tract is home to what is called the gut microbiome. This is an ecosystem in which billions of bacteria live. A healthy gut microbiome will thrive because the bacteria is helping digest food. The nutrients from healthy food then provide the building blocks for neurotransmitters, hormones, and a strong immune system, among other functions. If you eat something that has low nutritional value, you won't see as many neurotransmitters created; thus, you'll likely have a hormonal imbalance, and you'll open yourself up to disease/illness due to a weak immune system. Is this the body that God created in His image? A body that is prone to failure from within?

Not at all. What happened when the fruit from the Tree of Knowledge was eaten by both Adam and Eve (an important point that both individual gut microbiomes were separately affected) is the bacteria in the gut was forever changed. Obviously, because it was so long ago, science can't prove why that change happened in their minds, but we know it did.

What science has proven is the majority of neurotransmitters in the brain are actually created in the gut during digestion. It could in fact be that the introduction of a certain nutrient or bacteria found in the apple of the Tree of Knowledge stimulated a new neurotransmitter to Adam and Eve, which in turn enlightened their minds. Or did this nutrient or bacteria simply open up a neuroreceptor to begin receiving new information? Determining that won't be possible without direct input from God. In other words, ask Him when you get to Heaven.

God created in us a fail-safe system of healing, even though our once perfect human body was forever changed by the consumption of that one apple. What happens in your gut microbiome plays a significant role in our mental health, emotional health, and physical health. The issue we have been faced with is finding a way to tap into that healing system.

What I find particularly interesting is that the closer we get to understanding the connection between the gut and mind through science, the farther as a society we seem to be getting away from using that knowledge. The breakthroughs in nutrition knowledge seem to be squashed by the rising levels of chronic disease—the very same diseases that can be prevented by proper nutrition.

The scales are being tipped by one simple self-limiting belief that we all have. I know I've thought and even said it dozens of times (if not more) in my life.

"That could never happen to me."

It might be hard at first to see this as a self-limiting belief, but it is. It's not necessarily limiting you from achieving something, but it's limiting you from seeing the potential negatives. It's like when someone tells you to focus on the positive in a situation that didn't go your way. Their intentions are good. It's said in an effort to lift your spirits, but when we only focus on the few positive things that might have occurred, we miss out on the opportunity for growth. We learn more from our mistakes than from our successes.

It's interesting that Adam and Eve actually had a greater amount of knowledge about the spiritual world than we do today, but they gave that up in pursuit of worldly knowledge. In Genesis 3:8, the Bible says that God was walking in the Garden of Eden, looking for Adam and Eve. There is not much more of a personal relationship you can have with God than to be face to face with Him. In Genesis 3:1-4, we read the conversation between Eve and Satan, which again shows an up close and personal relationship. Adam and Eve were right there among the leaders of the spiritual world yet chose to pursue worldly knowledge rather than trust God's word.

Based on the way the story of the Bible is written, the eating of the apple from the Tree of Knowledge may very well be the first mistake ever made by mankind. A mistake that was made in the pursuit of a belief that there was more to learn. So what have we as mankind learned from that mistake?

I believe we learned that our own plans, just like Adam and Eve's, are not as good as God's plans. We also learned that temptation is a strong thing to turn away from.

God's plans are just better than ours. Anyone who has seen God work in their life can attest to that. One vision of the way God plans for us is to think back to when you went bowling as a kid. They would put the bumpers in the gutters, so that you'd be guaranteed to hit at least a few pins during each frame. We often see God's plan as the safe plan, with bumpers guaranteed to keep us on the path. But if you go bowling as an adult and use bumpers, would you feel accomplished? Probably not. You might even be called a cheater by your competition, even if it's just a fun game.

I tend to view God's plans a little differently. Instead of putting up the bumpers in the gutters, God allows the gutters to expand to an infinite width. He still wants you to get a strike, but those expansive gutters are both distracting and nerve racking. If we trust in Him, He will put us in position to make the strike. But when we begin to have limiting beliefs about how difficult the task is, we often fail. How accomplished would you feel, if you bowled a strike when staring down gutters that are five, 10, or 50 feet wide?

Mistakes, not learning from mistakes, and temptations are driving forces of our self-limiting beliefs.

When we make a mistake, we often limit ourselves in our ability to overcome that mistake. This is especially true when we do not learn from the mistake and eventually repeat it. Repetition of mistakes can solidify our self-limiting beliefs to the point where we begin to believe that they are a fact about us. Every time we think that same limiting belief, we wire our mind in such a way as to believe it's true, even if the thought is 100 percent false. This is where the term self-fulfilling prophecy comes in.

Self-fulfilling prophecies are those items that you believe with such fierceness that you will make them happen. Most of the time they tend to be more negative than positive in nature because they develop from our self-limiting beliefs.

Some examples of negative self-fulfilling prophecies:

- I will die from cancer
- I will never find someone to marry because I'm not worthy of love
- I will never get promoted
- I'm always late to everything

In contrast, here are some positive self-fulfilling prophecies:

- I'm going to win a state title by my senior year (That was something I told my mother after the state cross-country race my sophomore year, and I fulfilled that prophecy.) I'm going to own my own business someday
- I'm strong enough to beat cancer no matter what the doctor says
- I'm going to have the happiest life of anyone I know

If you've ever played golf on a course with a water hole, you have likely heard a self-fulfilling prophecy. I've heard guys say, "If there is water anywhere within 200 yards of my ball, it's going in the water." Even when the water is 200 yards straight off to the right from where they are aiming, sure enough, they hit the water. If you approach the shot thinking it's going in the water, guess what your brain does? It makes sure it fulfills your thoughts.

That's not to say you can go up to every shot thinking it's going to be a hole in one and actually achieve that, but you have a much greater chance of getting a hole in one if you think it can happen. And let's face it, if you said, "I'm going to hit that small spot in that lake that is 20 yards off the shore, about 125 yards north of right where I'm standing." you wouldn't be able to do that. But hitting the ball anywhere in that lake because you are fearful of doing it? It's almost guaranteed to happen every time.

Self-limiting beliefs tear away at our confidence. When our confidence is low, we can feel the next mistake coming. We also tend to more readily fall to temptation. Our belief that we can achieve that goal we've set becomes smaller and smaller. What's really hard to deal with is, when we start to believe our internal limiting thoughts, the people around us can see it. If those people are not the correct people for your team, they might not be as eager to help prop you up.

As a graduate of Texas A&M University, I can't help but relay a story that happens every baseball season during an A&M home game. When an opposing pitcher walks an Aggie batter with four consecutive balls (as opposed to throwing strikes), the crowd begins to chant "Ball five" and continues to increase the count until either a strike is called, or the batter gets a hit. In a game against Mississippi State in 2017, the chant got all the way up to "Ball twelve" before the pitcher finally threw a strike. The crowd in these instances is obviously not on the pitcher's side. The crowd is attempting to create a self-fulfilling prophecy in the pitcher's mind that he is going to throw another ball.

The biggest danger with self-limiting beliefs might just be that we don't want other people to know that we are lacking confidence. We don't want others to see that we don't believe in ourselves. The natural next step is that we put up a false bravado. We think we have to play the part of who other people think we should be, even though that's not who we think we are. We aren't confident enough in who we are to be real. We aren't confident enough to tell everyone else, "I don't think I'm good enough," or "I'm not the person you think I am."

Because of the lack of confidence, we are afraid of being judged as different from everyone else. The irony is that we are all different from one another. We are often afraid of being acknowledged for who we are, and without a solid foundation in our values, it's hard to stand for what you believe in. Those self-limiting thoughts we have try to prevent us from building something great out of our lives. Couple those thoughts with the judgement we receive from others, and most of us simply fade into the shadows of each day.

That wasn't the case for so many brave humans across history. Think about Rosa Parks. If you aren't familiar with her story, in 1955 during the beginning of the civil rights movement in Montgomery, Alabama, Rosa Parks decided she wasn't going to give up her seat on a public city bus to a white man. She knew exactly what could have happened by not giving up her seat, but she stayed put because she believed it was right and was arrested for the act of simply believing in her values.

Shortly thereafter, Martin Luther King, Jr. would rise up to become a leader of the civil rights movement. I have no doubt in my mind that he had moments of self-doubt about being able to accomplish his dream. But he didn't listen to those self-limiting thoughts. He coupled his beliefs with the courage he saw from Parks and pushed for what he believed was right.

We are taught to fit in with the crowd at an early age. In school we are taught to "act normal" instead of being allowed to show the free spirit so many kids have. And when that free spirit shows itself, society wants us to create a label for it so that we can lump similar free-spirit actions into the same group. Our differences should be celebrated, and we should not be demoralized for who we are.

Thankfully, the United States has moved beyond segregation. But that doesn't mean that we have conquered racism. Having grown up in Louisiana in the 1980s, I saw many instances of racism that would make one think that segregation was still legal. When I was in college in the mid-1990s, I shared an apartment my junior year with Darius, an African American friend. I distinctly remember him asking me one day if the Jim Crow laws were still in effect in Louisiana (The Jim Crow laws enforced racial segregation in the Southern United States and were overturned by the government in 1965). I told Darius they were not officially in effect because it wasn't legal anymore. But I did have to admit that I had seen several acts of segregation in parts of Louisiana when growing up, not to mention the racist acts I'd witnessed.

We had known each other for about a year before living together, so I don't think Darius was trying to see if I had a level of racism within me. But I do think he was attempting to relate the environment I grew up in with how I acted. In my recollection, I've never once acted, purposefully or not, in a racist manner or with racist intentions. That's not to say my actions were not perceived as racist by someone, especially an African American male who had a completely different upbringing than mine.

We are all different. While we all may have the same nuts and bolts (cells, organs, bones, etc.), we are all different because of how we think, the environment we were raised in, what we've seen and experienced, and the relationships we've had. We've all had situations go against us, but we've also had good fortune at times. It's the magnitude of the positive and negative things that is different for each of us.

Our self-limiting beliefs play a big part in how we react to each of the life situations we encounter. The stronger the foundation of values our life is built on, the more likely we are able to ignore that self-doubt. Once we have tackled the beliefs that hold us back, all we have to deal with are the fears created from external stimuli. That's what Rosa Parks did. She held firm in her foundation of who she was as a human being. She ignored the internal limiting belief that she should simply abide by an unjust law. Then she confronted the external fear of imprisonment and the physical beating that could have come from confronting racism face on.

When God created you, he gave you a purpose. He has also given us the ability to overcome self-limiting beliefs. The question then becomes: are you willing to fulfill God's purpose for your life without limiting who you could become?

Commitment #5: Add a 5-minute pause to your morning routine. Sit quietly with no distractions, breath deeply, and repeat positive affirmations about who you are and what you offer the world (saying them aloud adds to the effectiveness)

- Timeframe: Daily, starting tomorrow morning
- Vision: See all the positive outcomes that are possible when you believe in yourself

# CHAPTER 5

# Embrace Your Fear

*"Fear is an indication of what you should do,
no what you shouldn't do." – Grant Cardone*

Fear drives a lot of people. The fear of being shunned, the fear of being outside the group, the fear of something traumatic happening. Fear motivates people to act. While there are times where fear is creating a good action, most of the time this is not the case.

When I'm on a run down a country road and I see a dog start to charge through an open gate towards me, fear of being attacked definitely motivates me to run the other direction, and fast. In dangerous situations, fear is a beneficial motivator. This draws on the ancestral instincts to avoid getting eaten by wild animals. With most of society in the Western world living in highly populated, non-rural areas, these interactions with wild animals are now far and few between.

Our lives today have evolved to include fears from other humans, both physical and emotional. But it's the emotional fears that we need to do a better job of controlling. I've seen the word FEAR used as a few different acronyms.

Face Everything And Rise is one in which the objective is to face the obstacles and rise above them; to stand tall in your beliefs without being anchored down by someone else's drama.

False Evidence Appearing Real helps us understand that some of our fears are the results of our imagination. The turmoil we create in our own minds becomes so real to us, we believe it as truth. Having these situations happen can paralyze a person in their current life-state and prevent growth.

Forget Everything And Relax is one I like at times because we all need moments where we draw back from our world and simply chill out. Whether that's through a time of meditation or a getaway to a beach, we need those moments to recharge both physically and emotionally. That's just good self-care in action.

While these acronyms can help add some perspective to our fears, the reality remains that you cannot overcome a fear until you embrace it.

Growing up, I had a pretty strong fear of heights. The first time I realized I had this fear was when my boy scout troop was asked to usher at a Louisiana State University football game. It was my first time in the nosebleed section of Tiger Stadium. I remember walking out from underneath the stands to look out across the entire stadium. As I peered off and saw that I appeared to be standing at a higher point than the Mississippi River bridge in the distance, I immediately felt woozy. The troop leaders found a job for me under the stands by the concession stand until the sun went down, then I seemed to be fine watching the game. Whether it was an adjustment over time to the height, or the distraction of the game, that helped me relax, I don't recall. But I did get to a place where I could manage my fear of heights that evening.

There are two distinct events that come to mind where I've let my fear of heights ruin a potentially once-in-a-lifetime event. For a six-month period when I was eleven years old, my family lived in Edinburgh, Scotland. One day, we decided to hike to the top of Arthur's Seat, an ancient volcano that sits 251 meters above sea level, giving an excellent view of the city. It's also the site of a large and well preserved fort. When we started to get higher up the hillside, I had to stop and sit down because I was afraid. I sat there and waited for my family to make the trek to the top and then return back to where I was. I don't remember exactly how far up the hill I made it, but it was probably less than halfway.

The other event has now become an event that can't be repeated. During a high school choir trip to New York City, our group went to the observatory deck of the World Trade Center buildings, long before the attack in 2001. Because I was feeling queasy from the height, I remember sitting on the escalator with an open view of the street level far down below. Then, when we reached the top, I stood on the observatory deck with my back glued to the wall, terrified.

While I dream of taking my family to Edinburgh and climbing Arthur's Seat with them at some point in the future, a trip to the top of the World Trade Center has become an event that can't be repeated. It truly turned out to be a once-in-my-lifetime event.

I'm not exactly sure what the event was that caused it to happen, but, shortly after getting married, I overcame my fear of heights. You might call it maturity. What I believe happened is that piece of my brain that harnessed the fear finally developed enough for me to understand that I wasn't going to fall to a horrible tumbling death simply from being high up off the ground. I had much more control than it appeared. I had trust in the buildings/ground that

I was standing on. I approached my fear of heights with logic and understanding, and I now enjoy being able to look out from high places to see the amazing views.

Fear creates pressure. Often in today's world, that pressure is unnecessary. The pressure then breeds stress that goes unmanaged. Unmanaged stress breeds additional fears, and a vicious cycle is created. The more times this cycle comes around, the more difficult it becomes to break, and this is where your emotional health challenges and physical health challenges meet.

Poor health choices lead to stress and fears. Stress and fears cause a need to find relief, which is often found in foods that are high in sugar, which temporarily combats the stressful, depressing feelings with a rush of dopamine in the brain. Dopamine is a neurotransmitter that literally lights up our brains. An abundance of dopamine gives us an emotional high. Sugar is one of the quickest ways to increase dopamine in the brain. Unfortunately, dopamine releases that are predicated on sugar intake are short-lived. This creates an intense, almost immediate happiness or joy that is followed by a quick drop to an emotional low.

Anyone who has been on a sugar restrictive diet will understand how this works from experience. Days go by without any sugar. As a "reward," the decision to eat a sugar-filled dessert after a meal creates an intense emotional high. That high might last 30 minutes before the emotional drop begins. At this point, the thoughts of "Why did I do that?" or "I feel so gross now" or "I have no discipline" occur. While these thoughts alone may seem innocent enough, in combination with other self-limiting beliefs that are probably going on, it continues the cycle of fear. Fear that the goal of a healthy lifestyle can't be achieved. Fear that, because of one dessert, a healthy diet will never be possible long term.

As one client told me, "Once I make that decision to have one donut in the morning, instead of stopping there and eating healthy the rest of the day, I tell myself I have no discipline, and, since I already shot the day, I may as well eat all the donuts in the box." He fell for the self-limiting trap that he doesn't have the discipline to stop at one donut. Moreover, since he has no discipline, it doesn't make any sense to even try to be healthy the rest of the day.

What I told him to do about poor nutritional meals and desserts, is to make the decision and move on. Embrace the fact that you want to eat whatever the meal is. There are some extreme situations where one meal might kill you (poison, or if you have a rare condition/allergy), but in most instances, one meal is one meal. It's the compounding of meals without nutritional value that is unhealthy. What constitutes compounding is an issue each individual needs to discover for their own body. For some, it's one meal after another, but for other people and some foods, it could be having the same food type as far as 30 days apart.

I believe we will find out that being fearful of what you eat has nearly as bad an effect on your body as the nutritional value (or lack thereof) itself. This is where self-fulfilling prophecies play a part in your health.

If you believe that you are just an obese person who will never be able to be "fit," then you've written a narrative, and created a fear, that is very difficult to overcome. Alternatively, you could easily be an obese person who believes they are healthy in every way but outward appearance. This person will not only live a happier life because of a more positive outlook, but they'll actually begin to be healthier internally because their internal narrative is telling that story.

At some point, we all have to realize that each of us is ultimately responsible for where we are in life. We have to take ownership of ourselves. We can't put it on mom. Can't put it on dad. Not on grandma and grandpa. We have to say the words, "I'm responsible for who I am" and realize that it's the truth.

That means if you are an unhealthy, fearful person, it is actually your fault. Now put aside situations of abuse or manipulation where you were truly a victim of someone else's evil behavior—that's obviously an instance where you had no control. But most of us are not in that situation. Most of us have a healthy relationship with most people in our lives and therefore do have control of where we are in life.

Being in control of your life does not mean that you are not responsible for outcomes. In fact, it's just the opposite. You are 100 percent responsible, which means you need to take 100 percent ownership of the outcomes in your life.

If it's a great outcome, guess what? *You* are responsible for that. Enjoy it! Take ownership. Don't flaunt it in front of people—nobody wants to see that. But take ownership and share the enjoyment.

If it's a bad outcome don't blame somebody else. Don't blame a circumstance that didn't turn out the way you thought it would. Don't blame the weather. Don't blame your boss, your coworker, the client that didn't follow through on the promise that you thought they would follow through on. If something doesn't work out the way that you wanted it to work out, and you don't have a contingency plan to make sure that it was going to work out that way, it's your fault. You have to take ownership of it, then you need to repair that situation.

If it was a bad decision that led to a negative outcome in a relationship, you need to repair the relationship. It's your responsibility. If it was something negative that happened at work, you need to repair that situation. Presentation that didn't go well? Sales call that backfired? You need to repair that situation and not leave it for someone else; nor can you ignore it.

This is 100 percent relatable when it comes to your health. You make a great decision and, in return, receive a great outcome. But when you make a poor decision that brings a negative outcome—you get ill, you find out you have a chronic disease because you made multiple poor decisions—that's up to you to fix. Yes, you can seek help from others. Someone like myself, a health coach, maybe your primary care physician, or even a specialist depending on how bad the health consequence is.

Recognizing that you need help is a way of overcoming the false fear that you are all alone. None of us are all alone, unless we purposefully alienate everyone we know. The only way to alienate everyone is to listen to the fears in our head telling us all those self-limiting thoughts about ourselves.

Fear can be a motivator for your health, but it's the wrong motivator. Oftentimes, people who have a massive health scare such as a heart attack will be fearful of having another one. This fear motivates a change in their lifestyle, but it often doesn't last long.

When I have clients who've suffered major health scares come to me to get help changing their habits, I try to uncover what their motivation is. If it's to achieve more with their life, to be around for their grandkids and/or spouse, then I know they will likely be successful in making the change. If they come to me because they are fearful of going through that experience again, I know it will work for the short term, but they'll likely return to their old ways over time.

Just as time heals all wounds, it creates a void in our memory about just how painful situations were. The phrase "I forgot how much that hurt" wouldn't be a phrase we've said before, if we always learned from the pain we feel.

If your motivation is correct, you can achieve anything because the motivating factor will be larger than the fear factor. Why do you see people eating strange bugs on reality TV shows? Because they are motivated by the potential reward by a factor larger than their fear of the bugs or what health issues may result from eating the bugs. That's all it comes down to. Motivation over fear. Both create pressure and stress, and you can't live a purposeful, transformational, healthy life without pressure and stress. It's all around us.

Pressure and/or heat applied to a kernel of corn creates popcorn. The dried kernel itself is not edible. Post transformation, the kernel becomes a popular snack food. Why are you so afraid of applying pressure to your life? You might just come out more pleasing on the other side. Or you can stay on the shelf as a kernel your whole life.

Yes, sometimes the kernel doesn't pop. That's ok. Keep trying. Eventually it will. But if it doesn't, that might mean that path wasn't supposed to be taken at that time. Moreover, sometimes the popcorn burns when you apply too much pressure or heat.

There are several ways to make popcorn. It can be cooked on a stovetop with oil, microwaved in a package with butter, air popped, or popped in a professional, carnival-sized popper. Each technique offers something a little different. Air popped tends to pop more kernels than microwaving. Carnival poppers elicit an emotion you don't get from an air popper at home. Cooking on the stovetop takes time and patience. Then of course there's my wife's favorite: kettle corn.

The kernel of corn has no fear. But oftentimes we are that kernel of corn waiting to pop. Waiting to transform into the next stage of life we feel will be more appetizing. We have fear, though. It gets in our way. Far too often, we fail to transform because of fear. Sometimes we feel the pressure of life and interpret it as fear.

Often, we feel the pop coming and realize it's going to push us a lot more than we want it to. Just like I did going up Arthur's Seat, we stop in our tracks and try to avoid the transformation. Sometimes this allows us to avoid transformation altogether, like the kernels that never pop. Other times, we become the last few kernels to pop, versus the first few. It's great that both pop, but how often do you recall trying to avoid a transformation for as long as you could and then, once it happened, saying to yourself, "well that wasn't so bad", or "why didn't I do this earlier?"?

Whether it's for your health, your relationships, your career, or your faith, embrace the fear you are feeling. Get ready for the explosion of the pop. Transform into the person you want to be on the inside, so that everyone can benefit from the internal beauty you've been hiding all this time.

Commitment #6: Try something new that is outside your comfort zone

- Timeframe: In the next 7 days
- Vision: See yourself as bold and courageous

# CHAPTER 6

# Are You What You Consume?

❧

*"Too many of us now tend to worship self-indulgence
and consumption." – Jimmy Carter*

Before you can answer the question—"Am I what I consume?"—,
an inventory of what you are consuming needs to be done. This is a
systematic strategy for finding the root cause of the issue at hand. It
works no matter the issue or root cause, because you are not at this
moment looking for a solution.

The process of evaluating your life is always tough. Asking yourself
to be 100 percent honest with who you are is not easy. We all tend
to sugar coat our own lives while also overstating the inability of
others to understand our struggles. Being honest with yourself will
make this process a quicker one. Not necessarily an easy one, but a
quicker one.

Block out some time. It may need to be an entire day or weekend,
but the important piece is not how long the block of time is, but that it
is uninterrupted. Remove as many distractions as you can. No phone,
laptop, television, tablet, books, people, pets, etc. If you find it hard to
remove distractions to begin this process, it is a big sign that you are
well overdue for getting this done.

Once you are clear of distractions, take action on the first step. Define the outcome you want in every meaningful area of your life. Where do you want to be? Don't set a time limit on achieving it, otherwise you may risk thinking "I can never get there", but simply establish what you want the outcome to be; one that would bring you internal happiness. As Steven Covey said, "You must begin with the end in mind." Write down one to three outcomes that you would like to see in each major area of your life.

Now that you know where you want to be, take an inventory of everything that you consume. No matter what the health or life issue you are trying to resolve is, you must know what is feeding the root cause and giving you the output that's no longer desired.

Here are a few areas you will want to take inventory of:

- Food
  - Am I eating a healthy diet?
  - Do I consume empty calories each day?
  - Is my food typically fresh, or highly processed?

- Entertainment
  - Am I consuming uplifting media (sitcoms, movies, videos, gaming, social platforms) that fill my spirit?
  - Can I sit in a quiet room, or must I have background noise?
  - Does the media I consume have an underlying message that I agree with?

- Hobbies
  - Do I really spend time investing in my hobby?
  - Do my hobbies truly bring me internal happiness?
  - Am I only choosing hobbies to avoid confrontations with others?

- Possessions/Products
  - Are the items I purchase a necessity, or a want?
  - Am I utilizing the items I purchase for their given purpose, or do they simply take up space?
- Rest
  - Am I getting quality sleep and recovery?
  - Do I take breaks from work to relieve stress?
- Success
  - Is the success I achieve grounded in a proper purpose?
  - Do I only view myself as a success if other people recognize my accomplishments?
- Relationships
  - Am I vulnerable with those I'm close to?
  - Do I have 2-5 friends that I share every detail of my life with?
  - Do I interact with my close friends weekly?

Again, these are just a few areas of life that you could look at. I recommend you start here and then expand as you make progress towards your overall life goals. But try to keep it to no more than twelve major areas of your life to work on. More than that, and you can easily become overwhelmed to the point of inaction.

A key piece to remember—this is where honesty comes in—is to answer the questions as they are written. You're not asking yourself how much you're consuming, but whether you're consuming any at all—that is what could be detrimental. You might want to justify the consumption of a negative item, but that's not what this step of the process is about. This is simply listing everything out. Just taking an inventory.

You have to be brutally honest with yourself about the inventory of what you are consuming, so much so that you probably won't like yourself. If you are like every other human being, chances are high that there is at least one thing (but typically several things) you are consuming that is hindering you from achieving your goals and dreams. Identifying that item may in fact be easier for a close friend, spouse, or parent to do than it is for you to do. The reason is that we all rationalize in our heads how deep-rooted the issue is. How many times have you thought of the phrase "everybody's doing it" until you realize that not everybody is doing it?

The next difficult step is to be honest about your flaws and accept them as reality. Too often, we try to hide behind a false reality we have built up in our heads. Whether it's because we had a parent who over-inflated our sense of accomplishment, or because we have not personally experienced many difficulties in life, typically, our internal reality is different than what's actually happening. The strange thing is, most people usually perceive their internal "reality" as being worse than the true reality of their lives is; but because of the negativity they tell themselves, they don't realize how good life is.

Once you've got a full inventory, which again can take a full day or two to create, separate each area's list into what you feel are easily identifiable positive and negative influences on your life. This should leave a few items that fall into a grey area.

As I shared in the Introduction to this book, I believe in treating areas of our lives with a black or white approach. Remove as much of the grey area as you can. So, this step of the process will be difficult for those who have never spent time deciding what really matters in their life. People without defined core values—the values they hold as absolutes and influential in every decision—will find this to be a demanding exercise.

I will admit that I have grey areas in my life, but I'm also actively working to make them black or white areas. I'm also not saying it is a bad thing to have grey areas, nor does it make you a failure. But living with core values creates a life where decisions are easier, because you know what you stand for. Moreover, core values can and will be changed if you live with an open mind. You will change your stance on issues as you learn and grow.

Taking an inventory of yourself is difficult, but don't quit. This is the step of the process where you determine if you are going to act on your life, or if your life is going to act on you. Will you use this process to begin making decisions for the outcomes you want? Or will you simply make decisions to avoid the worst that life can throw at you?

What I have found is that people who do not complete this step are typically the complainers. I'm not saying you should never have a reason to complain. If a server gives you horrible service at a restaurant, you should definitely let management know by filing a complaint. It's the people who complain about everything that are the ones who often fail during this decision-making step.

When you are making decisions based on your pre-defined core values, with an understanding of the positive and negative effects of the things you consume, you assume a greater role in the outcome. While you may not have control of the situation, making a decision in this manner gives you control over your part of the situation.

If you want control, you must know where you are going. You can't get where you want to go if you are making every decision based on how the world acts upon you; you'll just end up where the world says you should be. You must have a set of core values, a knowledge of how positive and negative influences affect your decisions and a desired outcome.

The desired outcome comes back around at the end of the process. What is it you are trying to achieve? If it's a health-related outcome it could be to lose weight, improve blood test results, or lower your blood pressure. If it's a relationship-related outcome, it could be to spend more time with your spouse and kids without being interrupted by work.

There are a lot of coaches and leaders that will tell you that you must find your WHY in order to break through the cycle of bad habits and succeed. I believe your WHY is important as it directly correlates to your desired outcome.

WHY are you wanting to lower your blood pressure? So that you can reduce the risk of heart disease and, in turn, extend your life and the time spent with your family.

My issue with focusing on your WHY in each area of life is that the WHY by itself does not define the process of getting there. It doesn't address the root cause of your problems. Your WHY can be good motivation for staying the course, but that's really all it does. You must know your course, or as the Cheshire Cat said in Alice in Wonderland: "If you don't know where you're going, any road will get you there."

By now you have:
- Written down the desired outcome
- Inventoried the items having positive and negative effects on your life
- Determined your WHY

But there is something missing, right? We haven't talked about where you are right now in this exact moment. You listed what got you here, but where are you, and how far away are you from your desired outcome?

There are two very familiar phrases that are fitting to introduce here. The first is "History tends to repeat itself." If you don't learn from your past mistakes you will likely repeat them again. The only way to learn is to be aware of what is going on.

Something to keep in mind: when the world is acting on you, and all your decisions are reactionary to those circumstances, you are not typically aware of what you are doing. You are just acting in response.

If you've ever gone for a walk or jog and come up on a dog charging at you aggressively, you might have frozen in place, or you might have run. This is your body's fight or flight response in action. If you freeze in place, you are likely preparing for a fight with the dog. If you turn and flee, you typically won't know exactly where you are going, only that it's not anywhere near the dog.

In most cases, the dog is simply guarding his territory and sees you as an invader. If you went on the same route the next day to confront this same dog, and receive the same aggressive reaction, did you learn from your past? Did you not know that the dog was likely to be out and would charge you as you approached his property? Some people, while remembering that the dog charged them, would be in such a reactionary mode that they'd forget where on their route it actually happened. This is what happens when the world acts on you, and all you do is react. There is often no correlation between the cause of your action and your action. Therefore, you find yourself in that same situation more times than you would like to admit.

Another phrase that is key to remember is the commonly quoted definition of insanity: doing the same thing over and over again and expecting a different result. If we don't take an inventory of our lives to see where our decisions are being made, we tend to continue on autopilot, taking the decision making out of the equation. Unless you have already created a fool-proof plan for your life, putting your life on autopilot is as close to insanity as you can get.

You may have heard someone—a doctor or maybe a coach—tell you to listen to your body because it will tell you what you need. When you need sleep. When you need food. When you need water. All those different things. But listening to your body is just the first step. The more important step is asking yourself whether you are ignoring your body, or if you're actually following through on what you need.

Considering the rising rates of obesity, I would say that the majority of people in the developed world are ignoring their body. When you ignore your body, you are doing a disservice to the human race. It's not just a disservice to you. It's not just your body that's affected, nor is it your circle of family, friends, and co-workers. It's the entire world that's affected if you do not take care of your body.

So that's pretty harsh, right?

It's because we have the ability to create a ripple effect. There's a ripple effect based on what we do. It affects the people around you. If you want to test this out, it's simple.

How many times have we heard "pay it forward"? The drive-thru window at a coffee shop is the perfect example of the ripple effect at work.

We often see someone post a picture of a coffee mug on social media with a caption about how the person in front of them paid for their coffee. That's simply one random act of kindness. But does the person then share that they paid it forward by paying for the person behind them in line?

Ripple effect!

Not only did the first person paying for one coffee lead the second person to pay for the third person in line; but, when one of them posts about it on social media, it has the potential to then influence any number of people across the world to pay it forward with their next coffee purchase.

Now, if you eat healthily, you're going to be more productive. Multiple researchers have proven this. Providing your body healthy nutrients helps regulate hormones and neurotransmitters. When your hormones are balanced, and you have high levels of neurotransmitters such as serotonin and dopamine, your brain functions more effectively. A more effective brain means higher productivity—up to 30 percent higher.

Another effect of healthy eating, again due to the proper regulation of hormones and neurotransmitters, is that you are more likely to have a happier personality and, with that, a happier effect on other people. You're going to change the aura around you, which is going to affect everybody you come in contact with. The cashier you see at the grocery store. The pastor that you talk to on a Sunday. Your fellow "gym rat" when you work out. It's going to affect everybody you come in contact with.

It may even affect people you do not come in physical contact with, simply by association. You could be the topic of conversation between two friends because they are in awe of how positive and happy you always seem to be, which is a great indicator that you are living a life of positive influence. That's the ripple effect of your life.

The healthier you are, the more of the world you touch, whether you leave your city or not. It doesn't matter how far your physical body actually travels. It's a matter of your aura. It's a matter of your energy being spread, and that's what good health does.

It becomes a point of intentionality. Living your life with an intentional focus on your health.

The healthier you are, the more you love yourself. The more you love yourself, the more you're able to love others. The more you love others, the easier it becomes to love others. When it's easy to love your neighbor, you will be able to look past their faults and see them for their non-sugar-coated selves. And when your neighbor experiences your love towards them, it makes it easier for them to live a non-sugar-coated life.

So, I'll ask it this way: Is what you're consuming leading you to a life of loving yourself and others? Is it leading you to become a positive force in this world? Are you waking up each morning with a true understanding of your purpose?

If you are truly honest with yourself, these can be tough questions to answer. I want to challenge you to make a conscious effort to remove one negative influence on your life today. Don't wait until tomorrow. Don't wait until you've finished this book. Don't wait for January 1 to make some New Year's Resolution that won't last until February. There is no time like the present. Cut something negative out today. In fact, I'll make it easy.

Write down the most glaringly negative influence you are consuming on this line:

_____

I know I said to first take an inventory of everything in your life, but how many times have you read a book and never gone back to attempt the tasks recommended in the book? I know I've done that before—great ideas that I read about but never put into action.

Once you've identified that first negative influence, you need to take the next step. It may even be more crucial to replace that negative with something positive. If you don't, you very well may find yourself back where you started. So, on this line, write down the first positive influence that you will add to your life. Start today.

---

Let's say the change you want to make is to reduce the amount of video-based media you consume. First, you must identify a positive outcome you want in your life and whether or not the consumption of video media is preventing that positive outcome. Let's say you determine it is indeed a negative cause in your life. Maybe the positive outcome (or your WHY) you desire is more intentional time with your spouse and kids. How exactly are you going to go about reducing video time? What are you going to intentionally replace it with? Those are the two questions you must have answers for before you can be successful at making the change.

A 2018 report cited in *Tech Crunch* indicated we spend nearly six hours a day watching video based entertainment (https://techcrunch. com/2018/07/31/u-s-adults-now-spend-nearly-6-hours-per-day-watching-video/). I was one of those individuals with a hefty television obsession, until August 2017. At that time, I decided to start reading, both to break my self-diagnosed addiction to television and to grow as an entrepreneur. One of the key pieces of information I learned from researching successful entrepreneurs and CEOs is that the vast majority read daily and follow a dedicated exercise routine. I already had the exercise piece taken care of, so it was time to address the reading piece.

Before August 2017, I could count on one hand the number of books I had attempted to read in the previous 20 years, and I'd finished even fewer. So, to read at the level of some of the most successful business people (one book a week) was going to be a daunting task. To be successful, I would need to dedicate a specific part of my day to reading; so, throughout the remainder of 2017, I finished 18 books at an average length of 142 pages.

What is my television consumption like today? Well, the television is rarely on in our house anymore. We actually don't turn it on during the week until after the kids go to bed, and then only watch about an hour of Netflix or a sporting event. On the weekends, the television is on more, but we do still turn it off for hours at a time—something that would never have happened before. I'd always had the television on in the background. My roommates in college made fun of me because I would watch the morning ESPN SportsCenter reruns over and over (back when they showed it, like, four times in a row), simply because I was addicted to having the television on.

How has this changed our family life? Today we play games with our kids instead of sitting on the couch watching television. We go to bed at a proper time and get the appropriate amount of sleep. I even get up at 5 a.m. almost every day to read for 45 to 60 minutes before starting my day. After three years, I'm finally reading a book a week.

Best of all, Jenny and I have noticed we have less stress from no longer worrying about issues going on in the world. We don't get caught up in the little daily drama that consumes so many people in our society today. A lot of that drama, believe it or not, affects the way you see yourself and your neighbors. It helps to create that sugar coating on your life. It can prevent you from spending time alone in your own thoughts where you gain an understanding of who you really are. Instead, you start to become like what you consume.

Commitment #7: Schedule and complete a consumption inventory

- Timeframe: In the next 14 days
- Vision: A life where you recognize the negative inputs before they become a part of your life

# CHAPTER 7

# Layers of Misinformation

❦

*"What you are worrying about usually isn't worrying about you"*
*– Cleo Wade*

Question #1 - Is it possible that everything we have been told about our health is wrong?

Question #2 - Is it plausible that there are well respected, tenured organizations (governments, non-profits, and corporations) that have promoted an agenda that may not in fact be healthy for the human body?

These two questions may seem different, but they can have the same effect on your health in either a positive or negative way.

Let's look at the first question.

I would venture to guess that if you included the industries of health insurance, medical care, mental and behavioral health, nutrition, weight loss, fitness and exercise, and pharmaceuticals, the total revenue generated would be greater than every other industry—maybe even combined. Many of these health-related industries are multi-billion-dollar industries in their own right.

With so much money being spent in the health area, why is it so confusing for an individual to find the balance of a healthy lifestyle?

Remember the second question: Is it plausible that there are well respected, tenured organizations (governments, non-profits, and corporations) that have promoted an agenda that may not in fact be healthy for the human body?

Yes, it is definitely plausible; but, let me preface this next part with a warning that I'm not trying to promote a conspiracy theory of any kind. There are great organizations that have a mission to promote proper ways to live and succeed on this planet. However, there are other organizations that may have started with that mission but, somewhere along the way, were twisted by profits. And, of course, there are organizations out there that are simply focused on making a profit no matter what the consequences are to people or the planet.

Just like many of you reading this, I've had family members who have dealt with several different health issues toward the end of their lives. Let's look at how the care of an individual at the end of their life might correlate to how we interact with organizations in our daily life.

Medical issues at the end of someone's life often result in the need for different medical specialists. One doctor might specialize in cardiology while another doctor specializes in renal care, and so on. They are all needed because one root cause can lead to a systematic failure in one area of the body creating a domino effect in the other systems. If the cardiovascular system begins to shut down, it puts pressure on the digestive system, which can then lead to issues with the endocrine system, the nervous system, and so on.

What tends to happen is that the cardiologist will see the person and diagnose a certain issue, which typically leads to a prescription medication. Then the person is referred to a gastroenterologist for a diagnosis on their digestive issues, which typically leads to another medication being prescribed. This often happens with multiple specialists (depending on how systemic the health issues are), leading to multiple prescriptions. I've spoken with dozens of people who are genuinely confused as to whether all their medications can be safely taken together. Not being a doctor myself, I always refer them back to their doctor or trusted pharmacist with that question. It's a big question.

But is it plausible that one doctor prescribed a medication that doesn't interact well with a different medication the person is already taking?

The answer, unfortunately, is *yes*. That's one reason why most doctors ask you repeatedly what medications you are taking, both prescribed and over the counter. The vast majority of doctors see patients with the intention of trying to help. It's a helping profession. They genuinely care about their patients. But they can often be siloed into their own specialty. This can and does cause interactions in medications. The pharmaceutical companies know this, which is why any prescription drug commercial you see comes with a litany of warnings about which drugs cause adverse reactions.

Let me be clear again that I'm not saying doctors are bad or that you should stay away from all medicines. What I'm saying is that most doctors are specialists, just like all medications are made for specific symptoms. If you don't evaluate and speak up for yourself in regard to how you are being treated, you might get stuck suffering from misinformation. Withholding information about the drugs you are taking from your cardiologist could lead to an acute health issue due to drug interactions. Your cardiologist did nothing wrong—he was acting on misinformation.

An interesting thing has happened in recent years. The Western diet has started to turn towards an acceptance of plant-based foods, and several fast-food restaurants have recently begun incorporating a plant-based burger patty into their menus. However, over time, information has come out about the safety and health of the actual patty.

It's been revealed that it's not really the healthiest option. It may be the healthiest option on their menu, but it's still not super healthy because of the chemicals in it.

In truth, the fast-food companies are just trying to make more money. They are attempting to increase their customer base by providing options for those family members who are vegan, vegetarian, plant-based, etc. These companies are approaching their product line from the standpoint of "people are starting to want an alternative to our regular options." The majority of people wanting these new options may indeed be satisfied. What's interesting is that there is misinformation on both sides of the coin with fast-food plant-based options.

The fast-food companies (at least to my knowledge, as of this writing) have not once billed their plant-based option as vegan. They are simply calling it what it is: plant-based. Many people tend to assume that plant-based and vegan are the same thing, and they would be wrong more times than not. If a food product is labeled "vegan," then you should be able to assume that there are no animal products in the item. But just because something is labeled as being for a plant-based diet does not mean it's vegan. The true meaning behind the term plant-based refers to a product or diet that is mostly derived from plants. But it doesn't mean it's animal free.

Now if someone wants to go to one of these fast-food restaurants and eat a plant-based product, that's a win for the fast-food restaurant. Especially if that person would not have chosen to eat there otherwise.

You may be thinking: "I'm not vegan or vegetarian so what does this matter?" I get it. Let me explain a little more about why this matters whether you are a devout vegan or full-on carnivore.

There are two levels of misinformation at play here. Both are derived from misinterpretation and self-focused thinking.

First, let's look at the misinterpretation by the general public. Many people have been hearing about the health benefits of a plant-based diet. In an effort to try to become healthier and not be shamed by their families or friends about diet choices, people find the option of a plant-based, fast-food burger very appealing. When these individuals go out to eat with their families or friends that are not worried about what they eat, they can now all go together to one of these fast-food restaurants. The social atmosphere around eating is intact again. The issue, as previously stated, is that these options are not necessarily healthy just because they are plant-based. High fructose corn syrup is 100 percent plant-based but also a contributor to a number of chronic diseases.

The misinterpretation mistake is: plant-based = healthy.

The other misinterpretation is made by both the fast-food companies and the general public. It's that people who eat a vegan or even vegetarian meal plan are doing so only for the health benefits. While some do (I'm one of those health-benefit vegans, by the way), there is a large portion of vegans who choose to eat that way because of the treatment of animals, namely, in the meat and poultry processing industries. So why would one of these animal rights-focused vegans go eat at one of these restaurants just because they have a plant-based option? What these companies are betting on is that they would forgo their core belief about the treatment of animals in return for purchasing one of their plant-based options.

That is not the reality. The companies forget that these people are extreme in their core beliefs. They will not compromise those beliefs simply because a fast-food chain now has a plant-based option. These are people who are not sugar-coating their lives when it comes to food and the way they feel animals should be treated. While it may be considered extreme by many, maybe they are giving the rest of us a glimpse into what it would look like if we broke through our own sugar coating?

However, what *could* result from the plant-based options is for people on the fence about plant-based or low-meat diets to try these plant-based fast-food options. In turn, it could lead to broader societal and food production changes, and eventually to more affordable, healthier food options everywhere.

So here you have a set of companies that have done things the same basic way for a long time. They understand exactly how everything works in their businesses. They understand exactly how to make a profit. Now they're trying to grab onto people with extreme core beliefs about food. These companies know the people they can capture will be customers for life, because that's how extreme people are about their beliefs. If they believe something is correct, they will do it for the rest of their lives.

That's the level that you need to be at with your core beliefs. That's the level with which you need to be showing your core beliefs to everybody. Take the sugar coating off and let people see who you are. Let them see what you believe in. It's okay that it's different from what other people believe if it's what you believe in your core.

These fast-food companies never marketed their plant-based foods as vegan or vegetarian. They never advertised an intention to stop serving meat options. The issue was completely derived from a misinterpretation of the information. This misinterpretation leads to one more layer of misinformation that we must sift through on a daily basis.

With the technology available today, we are all bombarded with information on a daily basis. How each of us interprets that information is based on our current base of knowledge, how that information interacts with our core beliefs, and our trust in the person delivering the information. Of these, the only one you lack some control over is who delivers the information to you.

You've likely heard the phrase "put their spin on it" in regard to the way people deliver information. You could hear the same story from two different people, both of whom you trust, but because each person's "spin", or take, of the situation is different, you come away with different pieces of information. This is especially dangerous for people without clearly defined core beliefs. People's judgement and trust is then clouded by this new information because they don't know who told them the truth, since two people told them versions of the same story.

Police officers must be adept at gathering information from multiple people at the scene of a car accident and deciphering what truly happened, because, typically, everyone sees the accident from a slightly different point of view.

Without knowing your core beliefs, too much information at once—also called information overload—can send you into a spiral of indecision. We've all experienced this at some point in our lives. Heck, some of us are stuck in a constant funnel of information overload.

One of the most obvious times I can remember this happening to me was the attack on the World Trade Center in New York City. That morning I was working a delivery route, delivering uniforms, mats, mops, etc. in the San Antonio area. I happened to be on a military base delivering to the convenient stores, PX, etc. I remember walking into a small repair shop with a map, a few uniforms, and some shop towels. As I went to get my delivery invoice signed, everyone was glued to a small television watching the report of the first plane hitting the tower. I didn't think much of it, got my signature, and went on to the next stop.

It was the PX which called for a much bigger product delivery. After pulling up to the loading dock, I went to get a basket to carry all the mats in with. The store manager stopped me and told me about the second plane strike. He said, "Forget about us today, get yourself off the base now." I decided I should trust him and went back to my truck. As I left the parking lot and headed toward the base exit, several military Humvees turned a corner behind me. As I left the exit gate, it was shut behind me. I was fortunate enough to be the last vehicle to leave the base before it was on total lockdown. Right after I left the base, my boss called me. I didn't even get to say hello. He was screaming "Get off the base! Get off the base!" When he finally stopped screaming, I told him I already was off-base.

As I finished the route that day, which was another five hours or so, everywhere I went people were glued to their televisions for reports. It was as if business had come to a standstill. The amount of information coming in through so many different media outlets left many people stunned to the point of indecision.

Now that years have passed, I see the difference between the people that had had their core values defined and those that didn't. Those that did, took the news in and felt for those involved, but went on with their responsibilities. The reality for many of the people I interacted with that day, was that the attack in New York had minimal effect on the specific job they had to do that day. Those who were able to process the events based on their core values were able to move on with the job at hand. But it was a small minority of people that were not glued to their televisions.

Fast forward to 2020. With the ever-increasing social media influence, you can see layers of misinformation almost everywhere you look. Technology has no doubt changed the world. With that comes both positive and negative influences on our lives. Without a solid understanding of your core beliefs, it becomes easy to follow the latest trend while attempting to improve your life. But remember that our bodies—physical, mental, emotional, and spiritual wellbeing—has not changed nearly as much as the technology around us. Sure, there are people setting records in physical feats, accomplishing masterful artistry, and expounding on scientific discoveries. However, the vast majority of us are not that much different from our ancestors, except we live in a time with greater technology.

There is a common thread you will find from all the great teachers from history to today. Whether it's Marcus Aurelius, Socrates, Shakespeare, or today's Lewis Howes, Mel Robbins, Gary Vaynerchuk, and Robin Sharma—they all promote a message that it's important to know who you are as an individual.

You must cut through the misinformation that the world and others around you have to say about who you should be. If you are taking advice from multiple people without any of them being privy to your entire story, you'll likely get conflicting advice, just like the cardiologist prescribing medication that may interact with a gastrointestinal medication.

If you don't have a solid base-knowledge of your beliefs, you could find yourself consuming information that sends you into emotional turmoil; similar to thinking that plant-based fast food is healthy, only to find out it also contains unhealthy chemicals. Chemicals that send your health into turmoil under the guise of being good for you.

When you don't know what you want out of life because you haven't put your core beliefs and goals down in writing, you risk spending too much time on mindless activities such as binge watching television or over consuming social media. While these are not necessarily bad activities in small amounts, large amounts of time spent on them creates an information overload that will distract you from achieving your best life.

Once you understand who you are and how you want to be fed—physically, mentally, emotionally, and spiritually—it's important to evaluate the people in your life (both family/friends and influencers). Are they feeding you information that moves you towards your goals, or are they causing distractions?

Commitment #8: Identify something you believe simply because a "trusted source" told you. Research for yourself to determine if you truly believe it.

- Timeframe: In the next 14 days
- Vision: Constant learning provides wisdom that will be invaluable to future decision making

# CHAPTER 8

# Who is on Your Team?

*"When you run alone, you run fast. But when you run together, you run far." – old Zambian proverb*

Life is about relationships.

Relationships help us inspire each other. Just as we should be trying to inspire the people we meet, the individuals on our team should be inspiring us.

In today's ever-increasing technological world, true personal in-depth relationships are hard to find. You can see this in both business and personal relationships. Having a face-to-face conversation is quickly becoming a lost art. We all tend to be so busy with the things of this world that we've forgotten to stop and relate to one another.

Why are personal relationships important? In my opinion, Jesus came to Earth to not only defeat Satan through his resurrection, but to be an example of how we are to relate to one another in a truly personal way. Helping each other through the tough times, living our lives for God's purpose, and not getting caught up in the things of this world are all examples of this.

If you have a core belief built around faith, no matter what your faith is in, the only way to spread that faith is through relationships.

Relationships are important because we were made to connect with each other. However, it is important to note that social media does not provide this type of connection. Sure, I can be connected with someone halfway around the world via the internet, but it's not the same thing. A true relationship connection is where you can physically touch the other person because you are meeting face to face.

I see examples of this every day in my business. I work with individuals both in-person and via the internet. Clients say my in-person training sessions are more beneficial than when they do the workouts on their own because I'm present and with them. It might be stating the obvious, but the relationship connection when I'm there provides more support, more energy, and more intensity among other things.

When you are physically meeting with someone, you make an impression. Whether it's a first or hundredth impression, every time you interact in person you make an impression that is far more memorable than an email, text, or social media post. It's said that you leave a piece of you with every person you come into contact with. That's how you share your faith.

How much of an impression you leave with them is dependent on how strong your faith is. Let's look at sports fans in comparison. Fans of a specific team or school can get pretty over-the-top at times. I know I'm one of those fans when it comes to my schools. I've been so "obnoxious" with my fandom for Texas A&M that, one year, after beating the University of Texas in football, there was not a single day that went by that I did not wear a maroon shirt until we played them again. When I connected with people, do you think they got the point that I supported A&M? Most did. In fact, I had several people ask if I even had any other color shirts. I was wearing my heart for my school on my sleeve.

That's how strong and overly apparent your core beliefs should be when you come in contact with other people. There should be no doubt in their mind about who you are. Your faith should stir one of the following questions:

- "Why are you the way you are?"
- "How did you develop into the person you are?"
- "Can you tell me how to be like you?"

When someone asks you one of these questions, or something similar to them, that's your signal to share more details about your core beliefs. It's not your job to convince them to be like you, just to share with them why you are the way you are.

My wife, Jenny, used to get upset with me when we would go out to eat because I would always eat healthily, especially if we were out of town. She understood that, as a health coach, it is important for me to not just promote good health habits, but to live them. I know enough people in my community that it's common to see at least one familiar face every place I go. What would it look like if the guy who is always talking about healthy eating is seen eating fried foods or super sugary dessert? Jenny would tell me it's ok to eat like that on occasion, but my point in return was that if one random person saw me in the restaurant eating poorly, how would they know that's the only poor nutritional meal I ate all month, or even all year? Would their impression be that I'm a person who talks one way but does things the opposite? Your core beliefs should be the driving force of how you act both when you are alone and when you are with other people, no matter who they are.

M&Ms have been famously marketed with the phrase "melts in your mouth, not in your hand". The principal at play here is the outer layer of the M&M prevents the heat of your hand from melting the inner milk chocolate core. When we live a life with weak core beliefs, it is necessary to have that thick outer coating because, without it, we give way to whatever anyone else believes.

What we need to do is build strong core beliefs. So strong they won't "melt" when heat is applied, because then we won't need any protective layer. We can show who we are without fear of ridicule. We can promote what we believe in without concern about what other people think. Acting this way inspires others to do the same.

Once you have your core beliefs defined, it's time to find the members of your team. Don't do it the other way around or you'll wind up one day wondering how you became someone you didn't want to be.

Being firm in your beliefs attracts people who are also firm in their convictions, even if they don't necessarily agree with your beliefs. These are the people that will be able to call you out when you mess up, and you'll thank them for doing so, rather than being upset with them.

Think of it as if you are a recovering alcoholic. You attend AA meetings because the people in the group share one firm core belief that you do: alcohol creates havoc in your life and you no longer desire that lifestyle. That one belief may be the only thing that connects any two people in the meeting, but it's a strong enough bond to help hold each other accountable. Those are the kinds of people you need on your team. That one commonality provides enough of a connection that you would drop everything to help keep that belief intact for the other person.

You might think that finding the right people for your team is too difficult. It's actually very easy... once you know who you are. When you break through your outer shell and show your core beliefs to the world, you will begin to attract people that fit your team. Some of these people will be short-term team members, and some will be there for the long haul. You'll need both. When you are open about who you are AND surround yourself with others who are open with strong core beliefs, you will find that you grow in such a way that you begin to challenge some of your core beliefs.

This is a positive sign that you have the right team members. Relationships thrive when you practice active listening. Are you really listening to the other person to hear what they feel, or are you fake-listening to get what you want out of the situation? When you are solid in your core beliefs, you'll listen to understand someone else's feelings. You'll take the relationship to a whole new level, one that most people won't ever achieve with the majority of their relationships. It doesn't mean you take on the person's feelings or opinions as your own. It simply means you get to a level of understanding with them that allows you to see things through their eyes.

In his book, *Outliers*, Malcolm Gladwell shares the research completed by Lewis Terman in the early- to mid-twentieth century regarding an individual's IQ and how it relates to success in life. Terman followed children with high IQs until they were well into adulthood. He divided up a group of men he followed into three groups based on their level of success. In the C group were the 150 men who Terman deemed did the least with their cognitive ability. Since all three groups of men had relatively similar high IQ's, he found that the C group "lacked something that could have been given to them if we'd only known they needed it: a community around them that prepared them properly for the world."

The people on your team are the ones who have access to the locker room, the inner you, the core of your personality. Hopefully you have a few of these people in your life, because we all need them. Just as in my case, though, immediate family connection does not automatically mean you are part of the team. That's a spot that has to be earned.

Watching a high school or college sporting event can give you insight into how the attitude you bring to your team plays a big role in the team's success. When a team faces adversity on the field or court, do you observe the team rallying around every player, effectively lifting the entire team as a whole? Or does the team begin infighting; wherein, the more talented/knowledgeable players start arguing or yelling at the less skilled players about their inability to execute the plays?

Good teams are built with team members that don't assume they are better than anyone else on the team. The people on the team have one common goal: to win. To achieve that goal, they know they must all be on the same page. They can't be arguing about what went wrong, who's in charge, or what to do next. Being a good teammate means you try to see what the others on the team see and help them find a way to achieve better results.

When you are interacting with multiple team members in this way, you'll find out exactly how much you have to offer the team, your community, and the world. The team will begin to lift each other up, causing a ripple effect throughout the community as each member interacts with people in their circles of influence. As each team member stands on their own core beliefs, it will inspire others to develop their beliefs and begin sharing them. A thriving community can typically be traced back to a few individuals who stood up for what they believed in and were unafraid of any repercussions. The only way to do that is to be strong in understanding who you are.

Remember, there is always someone somewhere that you can teach something to. Never sell yourself short.

Have you ever seen someone take a branch of a fruit tree and splice it into another fruit tree? It's really cool to see this done with different species of fruits. Say you take a branch from a peach tree and splice it into a plum tree. What you get is a plum tree that will produce peaches on that branch. You might do this because you know that the peach tree is starting to die, so in order to save some of that tree and keep producing peaches, you might splice the branch into the plum tree. Now, the tree produces two different kinds of fruit.

Now think of your life as a branch. It is commonly said that you become the five people you hang out with the most. Well if those five people are the branches of your community tree, are they dying off? Are they productive or not? If there are no more peaches coming from those branches, it's going to be hard for you to produce the fruit you want to produce. It's going to be equally hard for you to have a positive impact on your community.

So transplant yourself into a group that does have positive qualities, a group that is being productive and fruitful. Even if they're not your typical group of people. You might be a peach, and maybe they're plums or pears or apples. But that's okay! The people in your life that are not being productive, and are not a positive influence, aren't the right people even, if they are peaches. Whether you see it or not, those people are holding you back from being who you potentially could be. Transplanting yourself gives you an opportunity to grow, produce, and expand without dying off.

I realize it seems easier said than done to leave your group for an unknown group. That's why it's so important to know who you are without any sugar-coating. When others don't just see but *know* the real you, finding the group that will lift you to new heights will happen before you realize it.

Growing up, I would not have characterized my relationship with my dad as close. It wasn't necessarily a bad relationship; it just wasn't a close one. As a teen, I felt like the world revolved around me. As an athlete with high aspirations I had a definite arrogance to me on the track, but I didn't think of myself as any better than anyone else off the track. I was not part of the "in crowd" in high school, though I like to think that I had good relationships with everyone in my life. Well, except for my sisters, but sibling rivalries are not always rainbows and unicorns.

Leading into the state track meet my senior year, I suffered a stress fracture in my lower shin. It didn't stop me from competing but did hinder my ability to train for the three weeks before the meet. I managed to qualify in both the 1600-meter and 3200-meter runs. Before the injury, I had run the fastest times in the state in both events.

Early in the state meet came the 1600-meter race. I placed a disappointing fourth, with the first-place time being slightly behind my best performance of the year. I was discouraged but knew I had to race in the 3200-meter at the end of the meet. When the time came, I raced well and won the state title. Afterwards, in the stands, my mom informed me of two disappointing facts. The battery on the video camera had died before the race, so she didn't have any footage of my winning run. I was ok with that. Then she said my dad had left to go to the LSU Baseball game with the intention of returning before my race. He didn't make it back in time, and now there was no footage for him to even watch it.

This hurt a lot. This was the first big issue I recall with my father that I could not forgive him for. I know it doesn't sound like a huge tragedy, and, in the grand scheme of things, it's not like he was physically abusing me. But it caused big emotional trauma to a guy who thought he was worth paying to see run. Being a 17-year-old kid without the knowledge I possess now, I sugar-coated my relationship with my dad from that point forward. I knew I would need him for financial help while in college, so I couldn't simply sever the relationship.

Seventeen years later, when Jenny and I began the adoption process to become parents, the issue of my dad not seeing my race bubbled to the surface. Here I was, planning to become a father, but I still hadn't dealt with this issue with my own father.

If you don't know the process for adopting children, one of the steps is an in-depth home study performed by a licensed social worker. This is not just a review of what your physical home looks like, but an in-depth look at who you are and how you were raised, the goal being to determine if there are any red flags. Going through the home study process was like a therapy session digging into my childhood. It brought up the good and the bad about my upbringing.

Like many of us, I wanted my kids to have a better life than I had. Even if my life growing up wasn't all that bad, I still wanted them to have a better one. I think that's a completely natural desire.

I knew that I would need to deal with this issue with my dad if I was going to be a better father than he was to me. At the same time, I was struggling with seeing God as a perfect Father when my perception of my earthly father was poor at the time. This is a common problem for men in today's society.

My pastor recommended writing a letter to my dad. A simple letter to offer forgiveness for harms that were done. A letter that didn't place blame or strike with anger, but attempted to remove the sugar-coated outer layer of our relationship to expose the truth. It took me a while to agree to write the letter, but I did it. Interestingly, my pastor also said it wasn't mandatory to send the letter. Sometimes just writing your forgiveness out is all you need to do, and letting the offending individual know that you've forgiven them isn't necessary.

I decided to send that letter to my dad. I wasn't surprised when I did not get a return letter, but I will say, when we talk now, it's easier and more enjoyable.

I'll agree with you that there is much more horrific trauma between fathers and sons, mothers and daughters. I'm not trying to make light of those with this example. We all deal with different levels of trauma at any given moment. But, regardless of the level of trauma, take the time necessary to work on forgiveness towards those that caused you pain. Don't let issues fester under a false layer of friendliness. Be intentional about forgiving those who hurt you.

In the end, my dad was allowed back in the stadium, but he wasn't back on my team. He didn't get to come into the locker room. Good, bad, or indifferent—it's just the way it was.

We are often more like God than we realize. Being almighty, He could have squashed sin right from the beginning, but He chose to give humans a chance. The Bible tells us, through the lives of several people, where God tried to help us, but our desire for sin always crept up.

Then there is this break right before the coming of Jesus. Hundreds of years go by without anything being recorded in the Bible.

I think of this as God's preparation phase. He was spending time away from humanity as He prepared to provide the ultimate pathway to forgiveness—the life and death of His son, Jesus.

When our relationships are strained by wrongdoings, our first reactions are often anger and the holding of a grudge. Once the anger subsides a little, we might let the person try to earn back good favor. This rarely works, especially if the person is not fully aware of how they've hurt us.

We begin to realize that the piece holding the grudge in place is a lack of forgiveness. The problem very well could be us, and our approach to fixing the relationship needs to change.

It's at this time we often retreat from the person for a period of time. The length of time away can vary but is usually correlated to how hurt we feel and how close we are to the person who we feel wronged us. The bigger the hurt, the longer we need. The closer the relationship, the longer we need. During this retreat time, we think back to the good times of the relationship. We envision what the future would look like if the relationship became whole again; not that it would be the same relationship as before, but that it would move forward with love.

We are preparing to forgive. Forgiveness is a tough piece of life. It should not be taken lightly. If we flippantly forgive someone, it's usually a sugar-coated message that still holds onto a core of anger. That anger will continue to break down the relationship even though the other person believes the relationship to be whole.

In order to forgive with meaning and totality, there must be a time of preparation. Are we ready to forgive? Are we certain we will not hold this action against the person? Are we ready to potentially be hurt again by this person in a different way? Are we willing to move on with a mended relationship?

Forgiveness that has been prepared for will typically last. Making a change without preparing is always met with objections. Shoot, even when change is prepared for, it's met with objections. This is true of any change—eating healthier, policies at work, morning routines at home, etc. Change is difficult to adjust to for most people, but that difficulty is made easier when proper preparation has been done.

In order to forgive wholeheartedly, we can't have any objections. Whether valid or not, objections to forgiveness will allow the original issue to keep smoldering at our core. Then we put a layer of sugar-coating over that issue when we interact with the individual that hurt us.

At some point in the future, many times without much warning, that top layer will be stripped away. If complete forgiveness has not been granted, the issue that has been festering at our core is shown in an ugly, argumentative form. This typically causes far more damage to the relationship than the original issue ever caused, and in many instances, after a festered core issue is revealed, the relationship is irreparable. There could still be a polite discourse when around each other, but the reality of a truly loving relationship is dead.

Here's the piece that is confusing for most to understand. How can you live a life without a sugar-coated protective layer but then only allow certain people into the core of who you are? The key word you must understand to do this effectively is influence. Just because we should live a life without a sugar-coated exterior, does not mean that anyone and everyone is given influential powers over our core beliefs. Likewise, you should not use your non-sugar-coated life to improperly influence others.

Commitment #9: Contact your 3-5 closest friends and ask them to hold you accountable to living free of sugar-coating

- Timeframe: In the next 7 days
- Vision: A future with strong friendships, lifting each other up, and celebrating great achievements together

# CHAPTER 9

# Failure is an Option

❦

*"Mistakes are always forgivable, if one has the courage to admit them."*
*– Bruce Lee*

I grew up vacationing at Lake Tenkiller in Oklahoma with my mom's side of the family. For decades, there has been a strong water-skiing tradition in my family. Papaw was the boat driver and ski instructor. He would always tell us, "If you're not falling, you're not learning."

As a kid, I didn't start to understand that saying until the summer after ninth-grade. Before that, I wasn't a good enough skier to not fall at least once during a session. Then, for a two-week skiing vacation, I managed to slalom every day and did not fall once. I recall having this major sense of accomplishment because I felt like I had begun to master skiing.

Once you master the skill of water skiing to the point where you are able to stay upright on the water under normal, easy riding conditions, it becomes very easy to not fall. You ride along enjoying the feeling of gliding on the water until you get tired and simply let go of the rope handle to stop.

Papaw saw it a different way when I started to brag about my ability. He reminded me of that phrase, "If you're not falling, you're not learning," basically telling me I might have skied well but hadn't learned anything in the process. I would slalom to the point of pushing myself just to the edge of discomfort and then back down. He called me out for staying in my comfort zone. Sure, I increased my ability some, but I didn't push to the point of true growth. I had some close calls but didn't have that big spill.

If you are not failing on a regular basis, you should ask yourself what's wrong. I know that seems backwards, but it's not. Should you also be asking what's wrong when you do fail? Yes, of course you should. That's just common sense.

What is not common sense is thinking that you're always going to find success in everything you do. You will fail at something every day, OR, you are not pushing your potential enough. That doesn't mean you will fail at every big thing you try, or that you can't have successful days. In fact, every day IS a successful day as long as you are breathing. Perspective plays a big role in success and failure.

One person's failure might be another person's success. It's all in the perspective that you take. Take Des Linden's 2019 New York City Marathon race as an example. Des won the 2018 Boston Marathon, solidifying her place among the elite women marathoners of the day. When she started the 2019 NYC race, she was definitely considered a threat to win. Des typically ran with an even-pace strategy, the goal being to simply wear other runners out with her endurance and strength. As the race started to unfold, she realized the weather conditions were perfect.

"It was a perfect day to take a crack at having a good one," Linden said after the race. "Even standing on the bridge, you could feel that it was light wind and when we started, it was at our back. Walt [Drenth, her coach] always says, 'If you can't run fast on a day like this, you might as well go bowling.' That's the conditions we had. It was a good day to take a big swing."
www.runnersworld.com/news/a29550839/desiree-linden-nyc-marathon-results-2019/

Des realized this might be the perfect time to try and push herself. You might be wondering how much more an elite runner can push themselves, but for someone who runs like Des to change the script and push the pace early was a definite step out of her comfort zone. Failure was an option.

"It's about trying something new," she said. "You're not going to have a breakthrough doing something over and over and being really conservative and really cautious. It wasn't about running stupid; it was about going with the flow of the race."

"The really good thing was I held it together reasonably well," she said. "It was good to test mental toughness and to know that you're not going to die physically if you do it a different way. It might hurt a little bit more, but the upside could be fantastic."
www.runnersworld.com/news/a29550839/desiree-linden-nyc-marathon-results-2019/

Des failed to win the race, finishing in sixth place. That's a failure, right? Yes and no. It was a failure since her objective was to win the race, but she also accomplished her fastest marathon in over two years, coming in as the top American female finisher, with the fourth fastest American time ever run on the NYC marathon course. Her race epitomized a saying we had on our college cross country team: You rarely run a personal record in a race that you win.

That basically means you have to fail in order to be your best. There is no way around it. Failure is a part of success. They go hand in hand. Oftentimes, you'll experience more failures on the way to the top.

There is a product that is carried in every home improvement store and every store with a hardware section, and you likely have one in your home right now that failed to work on the first 39 attempts. The scientists who worked on the formula knew they could develop it and get it to work as they envisioned. So they didn't give up after the first, tenth, or thirty-ninth failure, and, finally, the fortieth tweak to the formula worked as they desired and dreamed. That product is WD40, which stands simply for Water Displacement 40. The scientists desired to displace the effects of water, commonly rust, and it took 40 attempts at the formula to get it right.

I think you would agree that WD40 has been a hugely successful product for years. Did you know that the success ratio for WD40 was 39 to one?

39 failures to one success.

How often have you tried something 39 times, failed with every single attempt, but then kept trying?

Can you think of anything you've tried even 10 times, failed at every time, and kept trying as an adult? Most of us don't think in these terms any longer. We reach a point where if we don't succeed quickly, we give up. Our society has moved towards this idea that if you don't have success the first time at something, then you must not be meant to do that—a mindset that is completely different from in our years growing up.

Most kids find something they have a passion for and attempt it over and over and over until they master it. If you have kids, think about how many times they try to do a cartwheel. Or even better, think about what your life would be like as a parent if your child at one year old attempted to walk for the first time, took a few steps, fell on their behind, and never attempted it again. How different would your life be if your child grew up through their teenage years crawling everywhere because they gave up after the first failed attempt to walk?

Somewhere between adolescence and early adulthood, we tend to lose this drive to keep trying, especially if it involves a new skill. Part of the issue is the perceived reward is not grand enough for the continued effort. Instead of trying—failing—trying again— failing— and then trying again until we have success, we simply never attempt it or stop after the first failure.

How you address failure is one of the key ingredients to success. If you believe that you will never succeed because you stop with every failed attempt at something new, you will be correct. Very rarely will you try something new and have immediate success. On the other hand, if you enter into that first attempt knowing that failure is a possible outcome, you will be ready to give it a second try. Success is always just around the corner from failure—keep trying.

All too often it's the approach to a new habit, skill, or lifestyle change that is the problem; not our ability. Our brain tricks us into thinking that, if you change your diet in an attempt to be healthy and the scale doesn't move, then it's just not meant to happen. Or if you create a product and no one buys it, then it's not worth anything.

But I'm here to tell you the scale *will* move. You have to be disciplined long enough for the proper nutrition/exercise plan to work.

The product will sell. You have to spend time on customer discovery to find the people who need the product.

"Ask and it will be given to you; seek and you will find; knock and the door will be opened to you. For everyone who asks receives; the one who seeks finds; and to the one who knocks, the door will be opened." Matthew 7:7-8

I find this passage is used far too often by people searching for a better situation in life. Taking it literally would mean if you ask, seek, or knock for something, God will give it to you. Right away. The first time you ask.

While we understand through our prior events that this rarely happens in the literal sense, some of us still expect it. There are more times than I can count that I've asked for something very specific and not been granted that item or result. Think about it—if everyone who ever asked God to be an Olympic champion was granted that request, no one would have ever lost an Olympic event. Plenty of people who make Olympic teams for their respective countries don't win their event. Believe me, they want to, or they would not be competing.

It's like in the movie *Bruce Almighty*. Bruce, played by Jim Carrey, received God's powers for a short period of time. As a result, he had to deal with all the prayer requests from a small segment of the population. Bruce was unable to handle the onslaught of prayer requests and eventually folded by answering yes to every prayer. The result was reported in the news to be a record number of lottery winners, in which each ticket holder won just a few dollars and not millions.

What if we look at this passage from the Bible in a different way? What if it means that if we ask God what He wants from us, He will provide the answer? What if it does not mean to seek anything we want, but instead seek for Him, and we will find the wisdom He wants us to have?

I believe God wants us to be in unison with His vision, but since we aren't God, we will fail in our ability to stay on track with His desires. When we get off track, we simply have to knock, and God will open the door to reveal what He desires for us. That does not mean that we get what we want when He opens the door. On the contrary, we often get something we don't want, because His desire for us is to put down our selfish desires, move us outside our comfort zones, and live for Him.

It's those worldly desires that we confuse with God's desires. He blesses each of us in different ways, but we forget that when we see one of our friends succeed quicker than us. Jealousy is a strong emotion that results in us hiding our true feelings. We begin to sugar-coat our interactions with our friends who seem to have an easier ride to the top. We want to be happy for our friends, but internally it can create feelings of inequality. We begin to have self-limiting beliefs about our ability to succeed at their level, and this can create a fear that our friends will leave us behind. How often do you hear someone say, "Don't forget about me when you become a huge success?" This is 100 percent a fear statement, and when that fear grows, it can cause you to distance yourself from your friend. Now you are losing a person on your team, and the fear of failure begins to grow because the last thing you want to happen is another failure while your friend is finding success.

This could easily have been a factor in one of my closest, lifelong relationships. One of my best friends for decades is a doctor—we'll call him Frank. We have a very open relationship in which we share every detail of our lives in order to hold each other accountable to being upstanding Christian men.

After I was laid off from the job in which I thought I was going to retire, I felt called to start my own business from scratch. Talk about opening up an avenue for failure. Frank was there to help support me when I had failure after failure in trying to figure out what the heck I was doing with my new venture. After I found some traction and stability with the business, Frank began to have some instability in *his* employment which led to a job search. As we discussed his challenges, he shared with me the new opportunities he was considering. I remember at one point, Frank shared his concern over his monthly income because it dropped below $10,000 that month. I distinctly remember thinking to myself during the phone conversation, "I can't tell him that I didn't make ten-thousand dollars my first year in business. That will make me look so small."

I knew that was a ridiculous thought, because Frank already knew where I was at. Maybe not the exact number, but he knew that we were on different income levels. It was never an issue before, and, except for that brief moment during that conversation, neither of us had ever let it become an issue.

Our friendship doesn't have a sugar-coating to it. That doesn't just help our relationship, but it also influences how we relate with others as well. Frank and I are both better people because we understand how to share our failures with each other. Our accountability to each other opens the door for us to be vulnerable and humble around other people.

When we have that type of stripped-down, totally honest relationship with God, He will show us the clear path to what He wants for us. It's at that point that our life desires line up with His life desires for us. I'm not saying it's bad, and definitely not sinful, to have dreams and desires for your life. It's a matter of trying to line your desires up with God's desires. That's when your dreams flourish even through failures.

This is one of the most effective ways to deal with self-doubt. Following God's clear direction for your life creates a sense of confidence that truly can't be matched. You will act on the plan without the need for doubt, because the God who created you for a purpose is guiding you along the way.

Does this mean that because God is forging the path we will be able to avoid all failures? Nope. While God doesn't fail in His plans, we do. We still have a part to play in the overall plan, and, far too often, we screw it up.

Have you ever watched a baseball game? If so, you know that the pitcher and catcher approach each pitch with a plan. Whether it's a fastball down the middle, a curve ball low and inside, or a slider on the outside of the plate, they have a plan and agree on it. Then the pitcher has to execute his part of the plan. He has to release the ball with the correct force, at the correct angle in the pitching motion, and with the proper follow through. Not to mention he has to target the correct point over home plate. Then the catcher has to have his glove lined up in the right spot while watching closely and keeping ready to adjust should the ball not fly through the air to the pre-planned destination point. He also has to close his glove at the precise moment in order to secure the ball and make the catch.

Any one of these pieces of the plan could go even the slightest bit awry, and what was planned to be a strike could wind up being called a ball. Not to mention that the batter could latch on to the pitch and hit the ball.

Just like the plan of the pitcher and catcher, God has a plan He wants us to execute. Sometimes execution goes well and other times it doesn't. And sometimes Satan, unfortunately the batter in this analogy, gets a hit and ruins that plan. But just like that pitcher and catcher continue with the next pitch, we have to live our life. Right up until the game (our life) is over. If we are in tune with God's desires for our lives, no matter how many hits Satan gets in our life, we will come out victorious in the end.

Failure is not always that easy to deal with. There are two types of failure we must recognize so that we can properly adjust the plan. There is an "in the moment failure," like when a tire blows out on the highway due to a nail, and there is a "failure to prepare," like when I failed a test in college because I decided not to study enough.

In-the-moment failures are often more traumatic for our emotions. We don't see them coming, and they can shake our confidence. These split-second failures can cause us to have massive overreactions, such as when you have a tire blowout causing you to overcorrect your steering to keep the car on the road. It seemingly comes out of nowhere to derail your plan.

Dealing with in-the-moment failures can be stressful, but often we overcome these failures pretty quickly. We put the spare tire on, buy a new tire, and we are back to our plan with just a little hiccup to our timeline and our bank account.

An "in the moment failure" can happen in relationships as well. Let's say you are backlogged at work and forget to tell your spouse you'll be late for dinner. You failed to communicate a change in the daily plan; a change that could very well cause frustration for your spouse because dinner was ready at the normally prescribed time. If this is the only recent failure in the relationship, then it would likely be considered a fairly small issue. There may be an argument over the lack of communication, but it typically won't extend beyond that evening.

But when this communication failure compounds on top of several other recent communication failures, it begins to sour the relationship. Any positive actions of one spouse won't be able to overcome the lack of communication because internal emotions are boiling over with anger. This happens often when one spouse, especially the offended spouse, does not have a healthy confidence in their core beliefs, and this lack of confidence couples with their fears of inadequacy.

When in-the-moment failures of a similar nature begin to compound, you must ask yourself if it is really a failure of preparation. If you keep having communication failures with your spouse, it might just be because neither spouse spent time preparing to communicate in a healthy way within a marriage.

Preparation is key to so many areas of life. Frustration sets in when we realize that good preparation does not always manifest in success. It does, however, give us a much higher chance of success.

If your spouse realizes that he's going to be stuck at work past normal quitting time and calls to warn you about that, he's preparing you for failure of the normal routine. This allows you to adjust cooking dinner at a later time, therefore allowing the family to have dinner with everyone in attendance. This also avoids the potential for an argument over the issue.

Failures due to a lack of preparation are often easy to identify internally. When the failure occurs, you almost immediately get a feeling of where you could have done better.

Think of that baseball game again. If your team scout doesn't do a thorough job of gathering information on the opposing batters, it will be more difficult for your pitcher to avoid giving up hits. If several batters have a successful game, the pitcher may go to the scout to inquire as to why each batter seemed to have success hitting the very pitches the scout thought they would have difficulty with. Or, let's say the pitcher didn't prepare his throwing arm properly in pregame warmups. This could lead to failing to throw fast enough or on target, or to lacking the stamina to pitch late into the game.

The Boy Scouts of America have had a motto for decades: "Be Prepared." The idea is to be in a state of readiness at all times. Ready for what? To be ready for a failure, because inevitably something is going to fail at some point. You need to be prepared to jump into action, and when you do, address the failure then move on with the plan.

Knowing why a failure occurs is helpful, but being prepared for that failure makes it easier to fix and move on without dwelling on it. Dwelling on failures is nearly worse than experiencing the failure to begin with. When we dwell on our failures, it prevents us from making further attempts, because the emotional trauma of failure, no matter how small, is not something we like to experience. No one likes to fail.

Many successful people embrace failure, but that doesn't mean they like it. Instead, one failure simply means that success is that much closer to happening. Successful people envision each failure as attempt number 39, knowing that the success of WD40 could come with the next attempt. That's why failure is an option that we need to embrace.

Commitment #10: Make another attempt at something you failed at in the past

- Timeframe: In the next 7 days
- Vision: See yourself as someone who does not give up easily

# CHAPTER 10

# Focus Is Power

❧

*"The earlier you learn that you should focus on what you have,*
*and not obsess about what you don't have, the happier you will be."*
*– Amy Poehler*

"Damn the torpedoes! Full speed ahead!"

Depending on how old you are, this may or may not be a phrase you've heard before. It came about back when wars were fought in a closer range than they are today—hand to hand combat at sea, if you will. This statement is part bravado, part duty, and part focus. It takes some definite guts to head straight into enemy fire and complete a mission, especially when the incoming fire is unseen because it's underwater.

"Damn the torpedoes!" basically means forget about the distractions and focus on the task you've been given. It's a do or die mentality, and that's exactly what you need in battle. It's also what you need in life, because that's what it all boils down to either you do something, or you die without having done it. You can avoid the doing part (which typically leads to regrets on your deathbed), but you can't avoid the death part. It's coming sooner or later.

"Full speed ahead!" gives the connotation of power. It's impossible to divert all energy to a full throttle effort if there is a distraction.

You can't run all out in one direction if you are looking around to see if someone or something else is catching you. That's why I coach my runners to never look back. It doesn't matter what's behind you. Focus on the finish line and get there as quickly as you can.

That's why some racehorses wear blinders over their eyes. They can't focus on what's ahead of them if they see the shadow of another horse next to them.

Focus is power.

The next time you go outside, notice the sun. It brings warmth. Sunlight creates growth in all living objects. Too much sunlight, when focused, creates a power that can be deadly. Even on cold days during winter, focused sunlight can wreak havoc.

Sunlight focused through a lens like a magnifying glass can start a fire almost instantly, giving it the power to destroy at a moment's notice. That's what focus can do. It gives you power.

Power can be used for good or for evil. Sure, bad things can happen even if the intention was a good one. Light from the Sun causes growth—a great intention, but under certain circumstances, it can start a grass fire. Now if focus is power, focus can then be used for good results or evil results. Hopefully, it's obvious throughout this book that I'm suggesting using focus to achieve positive outcomes.

When focus is placed on good intentions, good things happen. When focus is placed on good and authentic intentions, *great* things happen.

Being authentic means you aren't sugar coating it, and placing focus on an authentic life is what builds communities. Communities thrive when they are built on authentic individuals coming together to promote the greater good. However, when someone moves into a community with inauthentic intentions, turmoil typically ensues. Drama gains ground and derails the progress of the community.

Drama is the biggest deterrent to focus.

Think about the last time there was an office drama where you work. How much work got done compared to how much time was spent gossiping about the drama? Drama slows everything down. We all know that, but it still grabs our attention. If the drama is even remotely related to something we care about, it will suck us in like a tractor beam.

A traffic accident is dramatic in nature. How many times do you drive by an accident and turn to see what happened? Even though we should be completely focused on the road in front of us, we are pulled by the drama.

For the past few years, I have attempted to drive by accidents while making a conscious effort not to look to see what happened. It's really difficult, but I suggest that the next time you drive by an accident, try to do so without looking at it, and you'll notice just how big your curiosity for drama is. If you can't help but look, maybe it tells you something about your ability to focus.

We often allow internal drama to build in our minds. Whether it's self-inflicted drama or created by our relationships, our internal drama wreaks havoc on our ability to achieve our goals. Internal drama halts our focus.

But to break through the drama, you have to be willing to be vulnerable enough to show the world who you really are. If you believe you are not necessarily the best person because of choices you made, you need to make peace with that, otherwise it's impossible to move forward. Allow that past drama to remain in the past so that you can focus on the future. Move to a place internally where you don't worry about making right or wrong decisions, but are focused on making decisions that lift people up, make a positive impact, and help the community. *Those* are always the right decisions.

However, decisions that lift up your community and the people around you may, as well as make a positive impact, be controversial. The decision may not be exactly what everybody else wants to hear. It may put you on the outside looking in.

If you're worried about what everybody else thinks, then your hard outer coating will get harder. You risk losing your identity, because you're constantly trying to fit into someone else's ideas. Block that internal message to blend in with the group. You'll be more open, more vulnerable, and you'll share more of your true opinions and beliefs with the group.

The more often you can do this, the more often people will see inside that outer layer. People will see who you truly are and know more about what you believe. You know what's going to happen? The byproduct of being truly transparent is trust. You will be a much more trustworthy person, in their eyes.

You are who you are. People need to see it. People need to know it. When they trust you, your life will change. Their lives will change. Quite frankly, that's how you find happiness. By living a life without that outer shell.

Removed from your shell, you won't have to stress about whether you did something the way someone else thought was "right." You won't have to worry about making the "right" impressions. You won't have to focus on who other people want you to be, and you can go about living today for what you want to achieve. You will be able to share your views freely, and your core values will shine, impacting others.

But not everyone believes in the same things. We need to come to an understanding that we are all different. We need to show a basic amount of love and respect to everyone that we come in contact with, and we should approach people knowing that they are going to be different than we are. By doing this, the amount of conflict in our world diminishes, the amount of stress in our world diminishes, the amount of love in our world increases, and the amount of success in our world increases.

But when we focus only on ourselves, the power of that focus drives conflict. We are not able to stop our train of thought in order to listen to what others are saying. When we fail to listen to someone's opinions, it often stirs up conflict. Allowing someone to be heard can be the most calming behavior you ever engage in during a stressful negotiation. It's about focusing on something other than yourself.

As a Christian, I can admit that we get a bad rap. There's a lot of "Christian religions" that focus on converting people, but the truth is the Gospel says we are to share the good news of Christ. That sometimes gets twisted into people thinking they should convert someone to their belief in the good news of Christ. That's not what we're supposed to do as Christians. We are simply to love other people and share the good news. Share the good things that God has done and is doing in our lives. It's God's job to then take that seed we planted and offer that person His love.

It doesn't matter to me if someone chooses to follow Christ or not. I get no satisfaction or joy from saying I converted X number of people to Christianity. My joy comes from sharing the love of Christ. It's God's job to do the rest.

Not all Christians approach their religion with the same attitude. We've become a society that gets offended so quickly and so easily, because we have changed from simply sharing "This is who I am" to becoming a society that says "This is who I am, and you need to become like me." But you don't need to become like anybody else. You just need to be yourself. You just need to understand that God loves you the way you are. You just need to understand that people will love you the way you are.

When you are able to do that, you can allow yourself to focus on what you believe in. That focus then becomes very powerful.

How does your health improve your focus?

Your mind and your brain are two completely different things. Your brain is an organ that works to direct everything that happens in your body. Your mind is your cognitive ability. Many people think that our mind is directing our body, but it couldn't be further from the truth.

If you think about it, you're not manually in control of very many things. 99.9 percent of the time you don't have to focus on breathing to breathe. You cannot tell your heart to beat, it just beats. You can't tell your liver to excrete enzymes or your small intestine to absorb nutrients—they just do it based on signals from the brain.

Brain health is critical to your overall health, and we all need to understand the connection between the gut and the brain.

The gut creates neurotransmitters, stores those neurotransmitters, then sends them to the brain. How you treat your gut microbiome affects how efficiently your brain works, and when your brain is not working efficiently, your mind cannot compute efficiently. The brain, the gut and the mind all work extremely close together.

In his book, *Outliers*, Malcolm Gladwell devotes an entire chapter to "The 10,000 Hour Rule." He details in several different scenarios how world-class mastery was achieved in an area of expertise only after 10,000 hours of practice. One of the neurologists Gladwell cites, Daniel Levitin, states: "The emerging picture from such studies is that ten thousand hours of practice is required to achieve the level of mastery associated with being a world-class expert—in anything." Levitin shares that studies have been done on people in all walks of life from all different types of professions, and the 10,000-hours rule stands firm. Levitin concludes: "It seems that it takes the brain this long to assimilate all that it needs to know to achieve true mastery."

What that doesn't say is how long it takes you to achieve those 10,000 hours. If it's continuous, as in you never do anything else except that single activity you are attempting to become an expert in, it would take almost 14 consecutive months. That's without sleeping or eating, unless of course you wanted to become an expert at sleeping or eating. An American with a full-time job typically spends about 2,000 hours a year at work (not accounting for overtime). Simple math says it would take five years of full-time work to become an expert at your position, assuming you don't get a promotion or change job skills. With that in mind, you can determine how quickly you become an expert at a subject matter simply by adjusting how much time you focus on it.

I've heard another avenue to becoming an expert is simply to read 10 or more books a year on a subject, for two years. Doing so puts you in the rare company of Americans who have done that much research on a subject. Especially considering most Americans only read between one to three books a year, total.

When you become an expert in a subject, it brings with it a certain amount of power. Not necessarily the power that can be wielded to make people do what you want, but it could bring on a management position, or the ability to generate income from helping people in the community. When you are considered an expert, people listen to what you have to say in your area of expertise.

If we take that 14 months of continuous focus and apply it to the human gut, what do you think we get? For someone who decides to move from eating the Standard American Diet (SAD diet) to eating a proper healthy nutritional meal plan, it takes 14 months for the gut microbiome to become an expert at this proper healthy nutrition. Given that most people struggle with the meal changes at the beginning or make very slight changes at first to build into a fully nutritional meal plan, it's safe to say it might take 18-24 months before their gut gets a continuous 14 months of healthy meals to digest. Do you think that might be one explanation why it is so hard for people to make a sustainable change to their eating?

Keeping focused on healthy behavior brings on the power to complete the changes needed for a life free of sugar coating.

Commitment #11: Write down 3 positive goals to achieve each day, check them off as they are completed

- Timeframe: Daily in the morning, starting tomorrow
- Vision: See yourself smiling as you go to bed each night knowing you had a positive impact on the world that day

# CHAPTER 11

# Trust the Process

❦

*"Sweat more in practice, bleed less in war"* – *Spartan warrior credo*

To live a life free of sugar-coating you must trust the process. For the past few years I've used that as a tagline for my business and also as a motto for the sports teams I've coached.

Trust the process is a simple phrase. There is no reading between the lines, and while it may be simple, trusting the process commands a high level of discipline, focus, and commitment. It also infers that there is a plan in place, and even if the plan you follow is faulty in nature but you trust that you will get results, something is going to happen. When the plan is a good plan or, dare I say, even the correct plan, great things can happen.

As an example, let's view trusting the process when you approach an intersection that has a four-way stop. The process, or law, states that everyone should come to a complete stop at the stop sign. Whichever driver got there first is typically allowed to proceed through the intersection first. If you are that first driver and follow the process by stopping, looking in all directions, and then beginning to proceed through the intersection, you would be pretty upset if one of the other drivers decided not to trust the process and failed to stop or yield while driving his vehicle straight into the side of your car. Even if no one was injured, everyone involved is now having a bad day. I've been in this car accident scenario before, and something like this can change how strictly you adhere to the process of driving, at least for the short term.

A lack of trust in the process brings all kinds of challenges, but doubt might just be the biggest challenge—specifically self-doubt. Even people who have achieved the highest successes the world has seen have doubted themselves.

> "I have self-doubt. I have insecurity. I have fear of failure. I have nights when I show up at the arena and I'm like, 'My back hurts, my feet hurt, my knees hurt. I don't have it. I just want to chill.' We all have self-doubt. You don't deny it, but you also don't capitulate to it. You embrace it." – Kobe Bryant, 5-time NBA Champion, 18-time NBA All-Star

Kobe Bryant was one of the best basketball players the world has ever seen. As a life-long Los Angeles Laker fan, I watched his career from start to finish. What is amazing about this quote from Kobe is that you never once saw him doubt his ability on the basketball court. Sure, there were games where his team was beaten and games where he was outplayed. But you never saw him doubt himself. For one of the greatest and most confident basketball players in the world to admit he had self-doubt, it should show you that you are not alone when you doubt yourself.

Doubt is a part of human nature. It can't be avoided, but it can be dealt with.

After being in a car accident, it's natural to doubt your driving ability. But over time, you realize the accident was a momentary breakdown in the process. Your doubt in your ability to drive diminishes with each passing day.

Doubt creeps in when the end goal of the process is not achieved. Did my plan have flaws? Was I simply not good enough to achieve the goal? Am I ever going to live up to my potential, or at least the potential everyone keeps telling me I have?

Self-doubt typically leads to stagnation. So much questioning is going on in your mind about why you haven't been able to be successful that you can't figure out what the next step is. Your ability to make a decision has become paralyzed. This is where you have so much doubt in your ability that you are unable to decide what to do next. Your fear of failure grows exponentially. You basically take yourself out of the game of life. You move to the sideline and let life pass you by.

Self-doubt is a feeling we all have. It's a flaw that came into being when Adam and Eve ate the apple. God doesn't doubt himself. Since we were made in God's image, I don't believe we were made to have self-doubt, but after the fall, we lost that luxury.

How confident are you about walking around inside your house completely naked, even when you are there all by yourself without your spouse to potentially criticize your body? Most people would never do that. Not because they fear someone coming to the door or seeing them through a window that's covered with a curtain. Most would not do it because there is a lack of confidence in their body. There is a shame, or doubt, about the ability to be totally free.

Adam and Eve didn't have that self-doubt. They walked around naked in the Garden of Eden until they ate the apple from the Tree of Knowledge and learned of their state of nakedness.

When our self-doubt rises to the level to which we are stagnant, we essentially become like Adam and Eve after eating the apple. They hid from God and were ashamed of what they had done. They had no confidence at that moment. They had lost trust in the process— the process where God said they could eat anything in the garden except the fruit from that one tree. The temptation created by Satan was so great that they ignored the process. Whether you believe the creation story or not, the interactions between the characters in the story are relevant to how we interact with those around us today. Every parent has seen this play out with their children. You tell them not to do something, then, of course, they do it but try to hide it from you. When you find out, there is a punishment that is enforced.

Fear, self-limiting beliefs, selfishness, misinformation, poor teammates, and thinking we will be an instant success are all reasons why we fail to trust the process. Sure, there are times in a competitive situation where failure occurs because your competitor simply did a better job. No fault of your own; they were just better on that day. But you must move your frame of reference away from wins and losses and towards being the best, most authentic person you can be. That's what trusting the process means.

Trusting the process doesn't guarantee an outcome, but it guarantees you will stretch yourself and grow.

"You grow most when you push yourself into the discomfort."
– Nico Rosenberg, 2016 Formula One World Champion driver

This is a great quote. If we stay in our comfort zone, we won't experience anything new. It's these new experiences that cause us to grow. Going outside your comfort zone is scary, but it's part of the process of growing both in your life and growing as a community member. While it can be filled with unknowns, trusting that the end result will make you a better person will help you overcome the fears, self-limiting beliefs, and so on.

Trusting the process does not mean you will avoid failure. It means you have faith the process will bring the desired outcome even when failure occurs. You'll have a built-in safety net that may or may not work, but it's there. Just knowing that failure is coming frames your mindset so that you avoid a huge emotional swing that could throw your whole life out of whack for who-knows-how-long.

Have you ever said something like, "I don't know why God gave me this ability," or "That's just always come naturally to me"? I believe these are clues to pieces of your individual process.

If you don't know why you have a certain skill, maybe this will help clarify it for you: I believe God created each and every one of us so we have special gifts and talents. Some people realize these talents at an early age, while other people ignore them. Some people use these talents to become financially or professionally successful, while others use their talents in volunteer capacities.

So, were we given talents just to be able to find individual success? I don't think so. I believe they were also given to us to help our society grow and prosper.

God gave us talents and gifts for the purpose of bringing other people into His family. He gave us our talents so that we could find joy in this fallen world. He wants us to lead by example, which is why He sent His son Jesus to Earth. He came to save us from our sin, yes, but also to lead by example, because our sinful nature is unable to abide by the law. Using our talents brings a God-given joy to our hearts and to His. This type of joy is an aspect of life that I believe every human being is searching for.

True joy and happiness are often byproducts of trusting the process that God puts in front of us. We can achieve short-term happiness simply by doing things we like that aren't a part of God's overall plan. But the eternal joy that lasts a lifetime only comes from realizing God's plan for your life AND trusting the process of living that plan out on a daily basis.

That's not to say that trusting the process is easy. It's not. It's also not an easy life to live. It's a life where God pushes you to show the world your inner self. He wants you to shed the sugar coating and show the world what lies beneath. He's given you talents and blessings that He wants you to share.

As a Christian, the greatest day I can imagine is the day that I die, because I will go to heaven to spend eternity with Christ. Now, the other side of that is to stay here in this world and get the most accomplished that I can. To do that, I must be healthy both physically and emotionally. I need to be able to accomplish more, be more productive, and be more efficient—that's what being healthy is all about. It is living for Christ, not living for a dollar, and not living for family members or experiences.

How can I glorify God through my actions? That's the question that I live with every day. Am I living my life to the fullest? If I do, He will bless me with experiences. He will bless me with a family that flourishes. He will take care of my needs; not my wants, but my needs.

However, it's important to note that my relationship with God is not bound by my ability to do good work on Earth. God loves me no matter what I do, the same way a father loves his children. When my kids do something seemingly out of nowhere that pleases me, like feeding our dog without being asked or treating a stranger with respect, it makes me happy, but it doesn't make me love them any more. Nothing could make me love them more, because that's just not possible.

Being vulnerable to the point of sharing your inner being is daunting. There is a confidence level that you must have in who you are. However, this confidence cannot reach the point of being egotistical, because that would tell the world you are insecure. We all know those people that are showy in their confidence in public but in private have a difficult time dealing with the internal issues of their lives. Their big bravado in public is a false identity that they continually prop up and maintain.

Without naming any specific celebrities, we have all heard stories of famous stars who are great to fans in public, but it later comes out that they are horrible bosses to their personal employees. That news always comes out at some point, and the longer it was kept a secret, the more shocking it tends to be.

When you approach every part of your life without sugar coating, there is no need to maintain a false reality. There is no need to worry about remembering what you told one person because it wasn't the real you. Not that it was a lie, but it simply wasn't your true feelings. When that happens, you have lost trust in the process of relationships. Your interactions with that person become superficial over time because they are not allowed to see the core of who you are any longer. Eventually, the relationship goes away.

This isn't to say that every relationship needs to last a lifetime. Relationships ebb and flow like the tide of the ocean. Some are meant to last longer than others. What you don't want to have happen is lose a relationship because you could not be real with the other person. As explained in Chapter 8: Who is on Your Team?, having the correct relationships at the correct time is crucial to your success. We can't go through this life alone. How we relate to each other in this world is a critical piece of every person's process.

When you have the correct people on your team, you understand how to use your gifts, and living a happy, healthy, successful life becomes a byproduct of your internal values. Trusting this process will allow you to be a benefit to more people than you can possibly imagine. You'll be an inspiration to people you don't even know. With the technology of today, you'll potentially reach someone living across the globe who doesn't even speak your language.

The only way that happens is when you trust the process of your life every day. It might seem mundane at times. The routine can get old, and the call to take a day off from who you are will be strong. It actually gets stronger and not weaker the farther along you get. That's why you must remind yourself daily to trust the process.

The more Christians I talk to, the more truth I find in this next statement. Satan will leave the lukewarm followers of God alone and go strong after the faithful, gospel-spreading Christians with all his might. That might seem to defy logic, but it's very true.

Satan doesn't need to worry about lukewarm Christians, because they are typically not actively spreading the Good News about Jesus. The people Satan does go strong against are the ones who are actively proclaiming the truth they see in Jesus. When you wonder why bad things happen to good people, it's often because Satan is trying everything he can to bring them down. Unfortunately for Satan, a believing Christian already knows that no matter what difficulties are faced on Earth, God has already won the spiritual battle.

This spiritual battle is being played out on Earth amongst us. That's why trusting the process that God created for you is so vitally important. This trust gives you the strength to maintain towards your goals. It gives you the courage to fight off temptations. This trust allows you to be vulnerable enough to show who you really are in your inner core without any sugar-coating.

Commitment #12: Have faith in the plan God has for you

- Timeframe: Always
- Vision: Arriving in Heaven and hearing the words, "Well done my good and faithful servant!"

# CHAPTER 12

# Honor Your Preparation

*Tomorrow's battle is won during today's practice. – Samurai maxim*

If you have ever tried to do anything outside your comfort zone, you know the experience of being nervous. Your stomach starts to churn a bit, and maybe your hands even start to shake. It's not just your mind that experiences nerves—it's a physical reaction. How big physically that reaction is often depends on a couple of things: how far outside your comfort zone you are going, and how prepared you are for the experience.

Bungee jumping off a bridge for the first time is likely to get your nerves moving. While I've never attempted it (I've overcome my fear of heights, but let's not push it too far), I've seen videos of plenty of people experiencing visible nerves before jumping. That's an experience you will get nervous about that you can't easily train for. The nerves are more associated with the bungee cord doing its job so you don't end up squashed on the bottom of a river valley.

More regularly, we see nerves in our daily lives in regard to our jobs, family communication, sports endeavors, and travel. Whether it's making a sales presentation, having an intervention type conversation with a loved one, competing in a local triathlon/road race, or driving across a tall bridge during a storm, we all experience different levels of nervousness every day.

Why do you think you get butterflies when you are about to do something outside your comfort zone? It's a reaction where different enzymes, neurotransmitters, and hormones are produced to prepare your fight, flight, or freeze response. Your body reacts first and tells your brain how to feel, and how intense the butterflies are directly corresponds to how prepared you are for the situation. If your gut is prepared for the oncoming stress, you tend to handle it well. If your gut is not prepared, you might find yourself in the bathroom with a giant case of the nerves, so to speak.

As a competitive runner, I see this response quite a bit before races. Those who are fully prepared and trained are focused and ready to go. On the other hand, you will see some folks pacing around the port-o-potties as they can't control their "nerves."

How do you prepare your gut for these situations? Eating healthy is a good first step. If your gut lining is healthy because you've fed it properly over time, it's less likely to have adverse reactions to an onslaught of enzymes. The second, but equally important, way to prepare your gut is to simulate the experience as best you can in the weeks before it happens.

It's obviously hard to simulate bungee jumping without simply doing it. But simulating a sales presentation is not only easy, it's highly recommended. I've had multiple sales and fundraising positions, each of which required role play after role play of how to take a prospect through the sales cycle. Alternatively, if you need to have a tough but loving conversation with a family member, you write down the things you want to say and repeat them in your head to make sure they sound both truthful and caring.

Simulating a sporting event such as a triathlon or road race is easy to do—you train. In the months and weeks before the race, you spend time each day training your body to be able to physically handle the strain the race will put on it. You may still be a little nervous at the starting line, but those are good nerves. Those are nerves indicating you desire to do well. However, being so nervous you find yourself sick to your stomach is an indication you aren't prepared either physically or mentally for the challenge ahead.

Proper preparation leads to an excitement type of nervousness. You are not just ready for the challenge ahead; you are excited to see how well you will actually perform. This is exactly where you want to be when taking on something outside of your comfort zone. When you feel those nerves coming on, change the narrative in your head. You are prepared. It's no longer nervousness… it's EXCITEMENT!

You might be thinking "If I've prepared for it, then is it really outside my comfort zone?" That's a great question. Logic would say that it would not be outside your comfort zone, but that's where you have to remember that human emotions and logic do not always end up on the same page. What you tell yourself in your head (self-limiting beliefs) can often overrule the preparation work you have put in.

Someone who wants to be an actor in a play because of their love of the theater might be able to be active in every practice, reciting their lines without a mistake for weeks, only to suffer stage fright when seeing an auditorium full of people at the opening night performance. That actor is fully prepared but allows stage fright to act as a limiting belief, thereby withholding their precious talent from the audience. When we find ourselves in this position, we must ignore the limiting self-talk and honor the preparation we have put in.

Now, having no nerves at all is not good. That's either a sign of overconfidence or a false understanding about what you are attempting to do. Simply put, you are never ready for what's coming if you are not at least a little nervous.

Confidence comes from putting the time into preparation and then honoring that preparation when called on to perform. Confidence is something we all need. Without it, we often drift through life without taking any chances. We will avoid tough decisions for fear of failure. We fly below the radar at work, just doing enough to get by but never achieving true success for ourselves or our employers.

Confidence can be generated in multiple ways. We can manifest confidence through our prior actions and successes. These can be simple things such as walking without falling down; or complicated, like catching a baseball on the run. When we repeatedly have success at something, our confidence in our ability to continue that success grows.

This is not limited to physical activity. Salespeople will generate confidence after making a sale. Managers build confidence in their leadership style after their team reaches a major goal. Students become confident from high test scores. Pastors gain confidence from delivering a sermon that is received well by their congregation.

When our confidence comes from our tangible past, it's easy to begin to rely on yourself. Your ego increases the more success you find. Thoughts about how great you are begin to swirl around in your head to the point where being successful in this area can define who you are.

I struggled with this in my athletic career, especially with running. For many years in high school and college, I defined myself as being an athlete above anything else. From my previous success, it was easy to do so. I was a three-time individual state champion and a member of several state championship teams. Less than 2 percent of high school track athletes receive a scholarship to a Division I university, and I was among them. Just in these few sentences of this paragraph, it's easy to see how my confidence and identity could be built on my ability to run. My wife even jokes that she would never have dated me in college because of my ego and inflated confidence.

After college, I stopped running. I didn't have a team to compete for any longer, and long-distance running is a lot of work. I wanted to take a break from the years of running, especially since I no longer had a paid-for training room to go to for aches, pains, and injuries. What happened next might seem all too familiar to many of you. I had to face the question, "Who am I?"

Confidence can come from someone you respect and look up to. When your parent, mentor, or role model tells you something about yourself, you tend to put more stock in their words. When a father tells his son he is great at something, he believes it, whether it's true or not. Conversely, if a father tells their son he is terrible at something, he believes that as well. Both of these scenarios can be detrimental to the child's emotional growth.

It's human nature to seek the approval of others. Our minds translate this approval as love for us. When we feel loved, we are more confident in ourselves. Someone else thinks we are great, so we must be.

Confidence can come from within. While this can cross paths with our past successes, our current situation can build our confidence for handling the here and now. The words you tell yourself in your mind—the beliefs you have about yourself—can lift you to new heights if they are positive in nature. When you see yourself in the mirror and have joy about your appearance, it builds confidence.

When you make a big transition in life like moving on from a sport that was a daily endeavor for a decade, it can rattle your confidence. With my running career, I made the mistake that many people make when they make a big life transition: I didn't prepare myself for the change in my lifestyle. I struggled to find a place of employment because I had little direction for what to do. I took a few short-term (two- to six-month) jobs before settling on a career path. Thankfully, Jenny stuck with me and didn't give up on me through all the ups and downs of me finding the new me (we got married in the midst of all that transition).

Looking back, I now know that I wasn't taking the steps of preparation seriously. It goes back to the lack of knowledge I had about studying. I wasn't preparing myself and therefore wasn't succeeding.

A big key to success is in the details. This may be contradictory to what some people preach—that hard work, integrity, determination, and passion are the keys to success. I believe all those are important, but it's the details that make success happen.

As a cross country runner and coach, I know that success in a race in late October/early November is built on the details of the training done in the summer months. How much base mileage you run during the summer provides the foundation upon which you race months later.

Bruce Lee said, "I fear not the man who has practiced ten thousand kicks once, but I fear the man who has practiced one kick ten thousand times." He's not afraid of the man with the perfect kick or the man who has 10,000 different single kicks to choose from. Bruce feared the man who put the preparation into the small details to be an expert at one thing. Do you see the correlation between the 10,000-hour rule I presented in Chapter 10: Focus is Power? 10,000 hours to become an expert and 10,000 times to practice one individual kick.

If you don't put the proper details into the foundation during your preparation time, success will be hard to come by no matter how hard you work. I'm not advocating not trying until everything is perfect. There is a fine balance between solid preparation and perfect preparation. When the safety details of the bungee cord and harness are ready, *jump*. Don't wait for absolute perfect conditions. Honor the preparation that has been put in place.

In softball, if the batter waits for the perfect pitch to hit, she'll likely strike out waiting for that perfect pitch. You have to swing the bat to get on base, even if the conditions aren't perfect. Babe Ruth is considered one of the greatest baseball hitters of all time, and even he struck out 1,330 times in his career, which is proof enough that you have to swing the bat to be able to reach success.

In every race I've run, the details of the training plan were completed, and the miles and workouts were finished. But I can count very few times that I've gone into a race having hit every workout time exactly perfectly. Instead of running eight 400-meter repeats at 60 seconds, I may have run four of them at 60 and four at 61 seconds. Not a perfect workout based on the plan, but still a very solid foundation. To not run hard in the race after that workout would be a disservice to my preparation.

Many former UCLA basketball players have recounted how on the first day of practice every year, the great Hall of Fame coach, John

Wooden, would teach highly touted freshmen and even returning senior All Americans how to properly put on their socks and tie their shoes. If you tie your shoes the right way, you get better performance. Your feet don't slide or move around. You lessen friction between your foot, sock, and shoe, which is extremely important should any of them get soaked with sweat. Tied correctly, your shoe won't come off during competition unless it's pried off.

Tying shoes is a basic little task most of us learn by the time we are 7 or 8 years old, but doing so properly is one of the small details in the preparation for performance. When you wear a shoe, you have confidence that the shoe is going to protect your foot. Tying your shoe correctly is setting a proper foundation for your shoe to do its job well.

That tiniest of details sets the foundation for success. Ask any construction professional about the attention to details of a foundation. There is a reason why the saying "measure twice, cut once" exists in the construction world. A slight variation in one detail, and a foundation might not set correctly. If not corrected early on, a poor foundation will lead to a substandard building.

Preparation is not just about building a foundation, though. It's also about knowing where to build. Where should you spend your preparation time in order to make the most of the life you've been given? It's a lot like living near the tropics, on an island, or in a coastal town in order to receive the benefits of the beauty of the area. While its benefits are great, you must be prepared for the dangers.

I have an aunt and uncle who live on an island in the Caribbean. Preparing for hurricanes is an annual event for them. Sometimes they have weeks of notice but other times it could be just a few days. For many months of the year, they must stay in at least a minimal state of preparation. Sure, they have beautiful scenery, beaches, and weather for most of the year, but one bad storm without properly being prepared can cause them to question living there any longer.

It's the preparation for what could come that gets them through the tough storms. They recognize the dangers associated with their locale and try hard not to underestimate them. That's how you honor your preparation, by recognizing how extreme things could get. If they prepared for a storm that turned and missed them at the last minute, they might be skeptical about preparing as diligently for the next storm. That's not honoring the preparation needed to show the storm the respect it deserves.

Are you preparing for the storms of life even though you may not have been hit with a big one yet? Is your preparation layering on top of the foundation of your core beliefs, in order to show the world your genuine self?

No matter what age you are, until you pass away, there is still time to live. Some of us are preparing more than others, but we are all still preparing. It's not too late. The world around you needs to see the non-sugar coated version of who God created in you. The life you have lived to this point has prepared you for something. Maybe you know what that is and you're already on your way towards accomplishing it, or you're too afraid to take the first step. If nothing else, after getting this far in the book, hopefully, you are starting to piece together who you are without a sugar coating.

Whatever your next step is I can tell you that you are prepared for it. Whether it's a big step or a small step, your life to this point has prepared you. More importantly, you likely already know you are prepared; it's simply a matter of honoring who you are at the core versus continuing to be who society wants you to be.

Honoring your preparation is simple in nature, but it's not always easy. I tell people all the time that eating healthy is simple. It really is. It's not rocket science. But it's not easy, because of the society we live in and the things we tell ourselves. Focus on your own journey, because that is what you are prepared for. As Lisa Nichols said, "You can't take the elevator to the top, it ain't nothing but stairs." The stairs may not always be easy, but they are simple. It's just one step at a time with a focus on getting to the top.

It's time to break through the sugar coating you have been living behind. The world needs to see you.

Commitment #13: Read books about the subject matter of your life's purpose

- Timeframe: Daily
- Vision: Having the wisdom and courage to help your community grow and prosper

# CHAPTER 13

# I See You

❦

*"We don't need you to fit in. We need you to stand out." – Jon Acuff*

In the 2009 movie *Avatar*, the world of Pandora included a human-like tribe called the Na'vi. The Na'vi use the greeting "I see you" as a way of saying they see the inner purpose of the beings and lifeforms they come in contact with on Pandora. They lived in symbiosis with the other creatures and lifeforms on the planet. The Na'vi used only what they needed, gave back to the land, and had an understanding of the relationships between all living things.

There is a lot that we can take from this movie. There was no need or reason for any of the lifeforms to be unharmonious with any other creatures. They understood their own purpose and the purpose of those around them, and no one benefitted unless everyone benefitted.

In a way, this reminds me of another group of fictional blue characters—*The Smurfs*. While the Na'vi were described as 10 feet tall, and the Smurfs are only a few inches tall, the two societies have similarities. The Smurfs were mostly named for their roles or skills. There was Papa Smurf, the elder leader; Brainy Smurf, the book smart genius; Hefty Smurf was the strong one; and Clumsy Smurf was, of course, the clumsy one. They each had a role that they were best at, and they lived up to that role to foil the evil Gargamel.

How do we as humans relate to these fictional blue characters?

First, we need to find out what our gifts, skills, and talents are, and lean into them. When we sugar-coat our lives to try and fit into a category that isn't ours, we are not only hurting ourselves, but also the ones around us. You are a gifted human being.

After we have an understanding of our own gifts, we have to share them with our society. It may not make you a millionaire or provide you with all the toys that society says you are supposed to have, but it will bring you a level of happiness that no one can take away. It also makes you healthier due to increased happiness and lower stress levels.

Finally, you must be like the Na'vi and see others for who they truly are. Not in a way that uses their talents to get ahead, but rather to combine forces for the betterment of society as a whole. Get people on your team that complement your gifts and core values. As humans, we get into a lot of relationship trouble when we interpret what we see in another person instead of truly seeing what they want us to see. If they can't show us their inner self, that's not our issue but theirs, provided we are giving them a hospitable place in which to share. When we approach a conversation without a sugar-coated motive, it's easier for all involved to show their inner self.

As individuals in a larger society, we need to allow people the space to be themselves, especially when their beliefs are in conflict with our own. Being an individual means just that—each person is separate in their own uniqueness. If we are not allowing people to be individuals, then we won't be able to see them. They will simply be a part of the crowd, just as a single tree looks to be part of the forest if you look at it from a great distance.

If you've ever dug up a stump of a shrub or tree with hand tools, you know it takes time. Each shrub or tree has its own unique root system. It would be simple to dispose of if you knew that each oak tree stump had five main roots shooting off at 30 degrees from ground level, all at the same distance from each other around the stump. Find one root, and you could easily find and cut through the remaining roots with a simple tape measure, shovel, and ax. But it doesn't work that way, because, as a tree grows, the roots go towards water and away from any obstructions in the soil. They grow around rocks and underneath concrete. They may spread out a great distance through the topsoil or dive deeper in search of water. Many times, especially in forested areas, tree root systems intertwine to provide strength and support to each other.

Often, we see the beauty of a big tree but don't take a moment to think about the intricate root system that keeps the tree alive. There is more to the tree, just like there is more to you. All the experiences that happen to you throughout your life create who you are. No one else has those same experiences in combination. NO ONE!

You may be thinking that some of your experiences are embarrassing, or worse. You may feel like you can't share them, or you'll be judged for them. In Chapter 9: Failure is an Option, I shared how we all fail. Sometimes we forget that other people fail, or we even feel that our failures are worse than other people's. Get the right people on your team who are willing to accept you for who you are, blemishes and all. These are the people who are striving to live a life without sugar-coating as well.

It's a simple concept but it's not easy. Going against the norm in society is never easy, but the more time you spend defining yourself, the easier it will become. Will you mess up? Probably... Nobody's perfect. Can you learn from your mistakes, become a better person, and help others through your experiences? Absolutely, you can.

When others see your authentic layers without any sugar-coating, you will begin to make huge positive impacts on the world around you and beyond. I know I want to see you. I want to see what you can do. The world needs a healthy you. We need you to be you!

Commitment #14: Create a list of 3 things each day that you are grateful for

- Timeframe: Daily before bed for 21 days, starting today
- Vision: Living a life where you spend more time acknowledging the positives in your life instead of dwelling on the negatives

# Conclusion - Faith as an Athlete

❧

*Do you not know that in a race all the runners run, but only*
*one gets the prize? Run in such a way as to get the prize. Everyone*
*who competes in the games goes into strict training. They do it to*
*get a crown that will not last, but we do it to get a crown that*
*will last forever.*
*Therefore I do not run like someone running aimlessly; I do not fight*
*like a boxer beating the air.*
*No, I strike a blow to my body and make it my slave so that after*
*I have preached to others, I myself will not be disqualified for the prize.*
*– 1 Corinthians 9:24-27 NIV*

Athletics has been a huge part of my life for as long as I can remember.
I first started playing soccer in first grade and learned to water ski just
a few weeks after my seventh birthday.

Work ethic and discipline are easy for me when it comes to sports.
My drive to compete (and win) is as strong as anyone I've ever met.
In my book, *Confidence Through Health*, I share how my passion for
sports translated into my field of study at Texas A&M but also led me
to my life's work. Faith has played a huge part in my athletic successes
and failures.

## Competitive Drive to Win

Thinking back to my early sports years, there is no particular situation or moment that I can pinpoint as the beginning of my competitive drive. It's who I've always been. I hate to lose at anything, from a fully competitive race to a friendly game of cards with family. Seriously, it's bad. There are games that my family members won't play with me because I'm a bit ruthless.

Competitiveness comes from a desire to win. The drive to be the best. That can only happen, though, by having faith in your abilities, knowledge, training, and discipline.

While I didn't always believe it, now I know my abilities are God's gifts to me. Each of us has been gifted in different ways. God's desire is for us to use these talents to build each other up. That may go against the competitive drive to win. In sports, for you to win means your competitor must lose. Only one person can win a race, or one team can win a championship. That's how sports are; life is different. Sports can teach us a lot about life— competitiveness, teamwork, drive to succeed. But we need to keep sports as sports and life as life. Sure there are winners in life, but there doesn't have to be losers.

As a kid, if I wasn't playing Nerf football, basketball, or badminton with the neighborhood boys, you would find me in my backyard kicking my soccer ball against the brick wall of the back of our house. I must have hit that wall a million times over the years. I practiced for accuracy and power, and I had to replace countless handles to the water faucet over the years. Towards the end of my soccer career, I added the goal of kicking it over the house and into the street, trying to completely clear the roof and front yard.

All that practice paid off. I was a starting defender on the team that won the U14 Louisiana State Title. We went on to compete at the U.S. Regional tournament in Ft. Lauderdale. I had the only assist to the only goal our team scored in that tournament, and while we won that game 1-0, our team didn't win either of the other two games. I had developed into one of the top defenders in the state for my age.

Looking back, I didn't put much faith in God's help when it came to soccer. I attributed my success to my practice, determination, competitiveness, and coaching. What ultimately grew out of soccer was my ability to run. I seemed to be the only guy on the team who never got tired while running. I might not have been the fastest in a dead sprint, but no one was running farther, or as much, as I was. In fact, my soccer coach actually asked my parents for a different "punishment" other than running for when the team needed to be disciplined, because I enjoyed running sprints (or longer) too much. Turned out, that would be push-ups. To this day, even though I do them almost daily, I still have a strong dislike for push-ups.

Naturally, the sport of cross country found me as a freshman in high school. I knew nothing about cross country, but midway through the fall semester, we had to complete a 12-minute run for PE class. The goal for an A was to complete eight laps (just shy of two miles). I remember finishing eight laps right at 11:30, and I kept going even though the coach told me I could stop. One of the cross country guys in my class, Stevie Maggio, came over and told me about the sport. He said, "I think you need to talk to Coach Boo, today." Apparently, Stevie had told Coach Boudreaux about me before I could find him, because he was ready to put me on the team.

Joining the cross country team took my competitiveness to a whole new level. While cross country is a team sport, it's also very much an individual sport. Me against the other runners, me against the course, me against me.

At first it was just that: all about *me*. During my freshman and sophomore years, I would just take off at the beginning of the race and try to outlast everyone else. My plan, though it didn't always work, was to take the lead early and hope no one could catch me. On the freshman team, that was a fine strategy. I typically ran in the top four on our team, which was also usually the top four to six in the meet. But as a sophomore on varsity, it was a different story. Our high school had (and still has) a tradition of winning state titles in cross country.

I remember that whole year running as the seventh or eighth man on our team. If you don't know about cross country, you are only allowed a seven-man team at championship races. Each and every race, Coach Boo, as we called him, would talk to me about not going out so fast, but each and every race, there I was at the half-mile mark leading the way. We ran the same course, Highland Road Park in Baton Rouge, for a lot of our meets. I bet I still have the unofficial record for the fastest 800-meter start on that course (only unofficially because it wasn't a record anyone kept).

Truthfully, I squeaked onto our state meet team having edged out a senior in our district meet I had finished most of the races next to. Coach Boo saw something in my potential. My running career was about to be launched.

It was the biggest cross country meet I had run in to that point. I'll never forget it. I remember it like it was earlier today. The gun went off, and hundreds of runners took off down the 400-meter straightaway. As I started to get excited and speed up, Tre' Hendry, our senior leader, yelled at me to run next to him. I slowed and fell in line right next to him. It was really weird going through the first half mile with 60-70 runners in front of me, but I did it.

As we went through the mile mark of the three-mile race, I was still close to Tre'. Coach Boo was telling us now was the time to go after the leaders. At that mile mark, our rival team had all seven of their runners in front of our first runner. It's really cool to watch the video as we go by the first mile and count everyone from both teams.

I went on to finish second on our team (behind Tre') and thirteenth overall. We won the team title, and my confidence in my running abilities was sky-high. Proof of that was me telling my mom that I would win a cross country state title before I graduated (I'll admit, I don't recall saying that, but she swears that I did). What a punk little sophomore I was, but I had confidence.

History will show that I did follow through on that statement my senior year by winning the Louisiana 5A Cross Country state title in 1991. That boosted my confidence all the more. I followed that up by winning two more state titles in track in the spring of 1992. If you want to see someone who exudes confidence, go talk with a kid who just won three state titles in a year. Maybe a bit too much ego, as well.

My college running years at Texas A&M lacked nothing in confidence, although the results were not as glamorous as in high school. Sure, I had some great races, but I look back knowing I never truly reached my potential. I allowed too many distractions into my life at the time.

Even though I had accepted Christ as my Savior during the summer after high school graduation, I was still a very new Christian. There were many times where I played the Christian role but wasn't really living out the values behind the scenes. Internally, I was often running for myself or my school. I failed to connect the dots between my physical abilities and the ability to be a light for Christ. I was a hypocritical Christian living a sugar-coated life.

Once I graduated from college, I let my athletic endeavors fall out of my life. I stopped training/competing and became a weekend warrior. I was like many other former athletes—I simply moved away from my passion and God-given abilities to pursue the next step in life, as the world says we are supposed to.

During my internship in the last semester of college, I met my future wife, Jenny. As we began dating, we deduced that we had several classes together at A&M but had never spoken to each other as we'd both been in other relationships. Interestingly enough, even without speaking to each other, she'd picked up on my overabundance of confidence.

When I "retired" from competitive sports, the ego was put up on a shelf. I still had a competitive drive but nothing else brought out the confidence like racing. In married life, I began to grow as a Christian. With the help of my wife and leaders at our church, I began to understand how to give control of my life to God. This is an extremely difficult thing for us to do as humans because each of us is born with the need to be in control. It's a desire that's so basic it drives babies to cry when they need something. Control drives almost every action we make unless we are actively communicating with God about what His desires are; even then, it's difficult.

As I gave more and more control to God, I found it difficult to ignore His call on my life. After years of corporate and non-profit jobs, I turned back to my God-given abilities and passions—health, fitness, wellness, and sports.

As a lead-by-example kind of guy, I knew the first thing I had to do: get back in shape. Not necessarily in uber-competitive shape, but I had to look the part of a healthy, fit person. On August 1, 2015, at my heaviest ever, 188 pounds, we bought a stationary bike and I began riding to get in shape. Yes, I know 188 pounds does not seem earth-crumblingly huge, but for my height and build, my healthy weight is 145 pounds.

It wasn't easy to get back into shape after years away from athletic activity, but the focus to do so was easy. Letting God take control, following His lead, and keeping my focus on what He wanted from me every day made the lifestyle switch easy.

In early 2016, after losing an initial 20 pounds, I launched my business, All In Health and Wellness. I began helping people with all areas of health, fitness, nutrition, and wellness.

To this day, I begin waking every day with a devotional then ask God to use me for His purpose. Next, I either exercise or take our kids to school, and then exercise. The Bible states that we are supposed to give back to God from our first fruits. While most people will interpret this to mean financial giving, I also see it as giving back to Him from the gifts He has given us. He's given me the gift of running; therefore, I run early in the day as a gift to Him—totally not the motivation I had for running when I was in high school or college.

As I started to get back into shape, God put it in my heart to race again, and this time, I would race for Him to bring Him glory, not me. As I planned out which race to tackle, my immediate thoughts went to going for a much longer distance, because I thought "being older means I'm now slow."

After choosing the 2016 Bryan/College Station Marathon, I began training more seriously, rather than simply for good health. On July

14, 2016 (after already paying to enter the race), I went water skiing on our family vacation. I was on trick skis on what was to be the last ski pass of the morning before brunch. As I approached the water in front of our campsite, I prepared for a wake helicopter. In this maneuver, you start with the rope behind your back, you jump the wake, and then you spin 360 degrees in the air before landing and riding off. I'd never before attempted the trick, much less completed it.

As my brother-in-law stated, my right leg went around 360 but my left made it about 310. The ski stuck into the water at an angle that caused me to faceplant in a fraction of a second. I remember screaming under water as I had instant pain in my left leg. When I pulled my head out of the water, I lifted my leg to see what it looked like. In that instance, I knew my knee was jacked up because I had to push the head of the tibia back into place. Being an exercise physiologist, I knew my MCL was shredded. I initially thought I had torn up my ankle as well, but, thankfully, that was just pain from the ski being twisted on my foot.

A few days later, the MRI results revealed that I did indeed have a third-degree tear of my MCL, but the bigger issue was the completely ruptured PCL. I knew I could recover and run again from an MCL, but a PCL brought a whole new concern.

The surgeon I saw said I didn't need surgery (praise God) but shouldn't even think about running until January. I told him that wasn't going to work because God told me to run the BCS Marathon in December, a month before the doctor's recommended starting date. He shook his head and said, "Don't be crazy, that's not possible." With lots of prayer, I still heard God saying, "Run the race."

Having at least a little sense, I contacted the race registration team and dropped down from the marathon to the half-marathon. Even though the race would be shorter, I only had five months to rehab and train. I started doing everything I knew to do at home to begin the rehabilitation process.

When I went in for my initial physical therapy evaluation, I literally scared the therapist. First, I showed up in my running attire: super short shorts and running shoes. Then, when he asked what I expected to achieve from therapy, I responded, "To run a half-marathon in December." His response was simple and honest, "I don't think I can be your therapist." He went on to say he'd never competed in sports and would not be able to keep up with that kind of competitive drive. I greatly appreciated his honest response.

He did the evaluation and then passed me on to Dr. Celeste Quiroz for rehab. I know a lot of physical therapists from being a patient and as colleagues in fitness, and Celeste is one of the best. Not just because she did a great job handling my rehab, but because she listened and adjusted the plan for rehab as necessary without too much concern about what the surgeon said. I don't mean to say she went all rogue or against protocol, but what she did do was allow me to progress based on what the knee was physically able to handle; not based on a 5 minute office visit with the surgeon every six weeks.

Even though it was several years ago, I bet I could still do an impression of her face each visit when I would tell her what I accomplished at home during my personal therapy time. It was a look of both amazement, concern, and "you're insane," often followed with a statement to the effect, "Well, I may need to change our plan for today, because you've surpassed what I wanted to try."

I specifically remember one Wednesday night where I had taken our children to church for their Wednesday night activities. Instead of driving all the way home to then turning right around and coming back to pick them up, I decided to stay at the church. I found a quiet spot to pray a little, and I heard God tell me to attempt walking up the stairs. I hadn't done stairs without pretty serious help since the accident, and, keep in mind, I was wearing a brace on my knee at all times.

I looked around as if to see if anyone would stop me, which of course no one would have, then I got up and took off up the stairs. No using the hand railing, just stair after stair. I made it to the top without any issues. But I knew that going down would be more difficult. Without a PCL, there is nothing to help stabilize the lower leg as it goes back, and, therefore, it basically sticks to the step. But onward and downward, I went, and I took the first flight without too much issue. Did I just leave it at one and say it was done? Nope. 30 flights later, I did cause some attention when a few people asked if I was supposed to be doing stairs. I simply said, "Well, it doesn't hurt."

The next day, when I showed up at therapy, Celeste asked me what I thought about attempting stairs after the warmup. I smiled really big and told her I had completed 30 flights the night before. She looked at me like "of course you did." She commented that it could have been really bad because if my foot placement was off, the knee could have had undue strain in the wrong area which could have caused a set-back. I confidently said, "Let's go do some now, so you can see." After one flight up and down with her staring at my knee, I looked at her, and she looked at me. Then she matter-of-factly said, "You've got that down, on to the next thing." I never asked her, but I think it was at that moment that she realized I was going to push her just as much as she was pushing my knee. That's also the session where I could see her start to believe that I could actually run the race in December.

Even though we never talked about it specifically, I could tell by the way she spoke that she believed in God. I do believe that God strengthened her belief through my journey. I would regularly remind her that God told me to run the upcoming race, so I had to be ready.

The next hurdle after stairs was to actually jog on a treadmill. This happened on September 23. I remember Celeste and I were both nervous. It was sort of the make-or-break moment of the goal to run the race. Before the injury, I was routinely running anywhere from 30 minutes to an hour or more at a time at around a seven-minute mile pace. This first jog was a very managed, carefully scrutinized THREE minutes at 8:45-minute-mile pace.

I thanked God when getting off that treadmill after what seemed like an extra-long three minutes. Not because it was tiring, but because I was watching Celeste focus so intently on my knee's movement. Now that the first jog was successfully in the books, it was time to see what the surgeon said. Of course, he wasn't too pleased and was still against any running outside on uneven ground before January.

I was a bit deflated after that visit with the surgeon. I contacted my primary care doctor, who understood my passion for running, and asked if I could get a referral for a second opinion. He said he was glad to provide one and asked if I had a doctor in mind. I told him the only doctor I wanted to see, if possible, was Dr. J.P. Bramhall in College Station. Dr. Bramhall was the team doctor for A&M when I was running in college and is still there today. I knew he spent a year in Alabama with Dr. James Andrews, who is regarded as the top sports orthopedic surgeon in the country. Dr. Bramhall knows sports injuries. If he told me to quit on my goal of racing in December, then I would have no choice but to stop.

On October 10, we made the drive to College Station to see Dr. Bramhall. I'll never forget when he walked in and asked why I was there. I told him I wanted to run the half-marathon in December, but the other surgeon had ruled against it. He asked if it hurt to run with the brace on, and I honestly replied that it did not. He replied, "Then run the race."

Jenny and I looked at each other. She had this look of "great … oh crap" on her face. I think she knew the competitiveness was about to be ratcheted up a notch. From that day, I only had nine and a half weeks to train for the race.

I continued physical therapy for a few more weeks before clearing the point where insurance would not pay for any more sessions. Celeste and I continued to push my knee harder and harder. I remember one day during the second to last week of therapy where she finally created an hourlong therapy session that caused me to ask for a break. To that point, it was always me completing the prescribed task and asking for more. She had this big smile of accomplishment on her face. She'd finally broken me, but in a good way.

In the final 5 weeks prior to the race, I averaged just 17 miles a week. That's barely more than the 13.1 miles of a half-marathon. But, as I've told anyone who has asked about running a half-marathon, you only need to be able to run half the distance in training to be able to simply finish. While my pre-injury goal was to do more than finish, finishing was the only thing on my mind as I toed the line on Sunday, December 11, 2016, to race 13.1 miles.

I felt as if I'd started the race at a comfortable pace. I purposefully did not wear a watch, because I didn't want to be constantly focused on time; the goal was to finish and keep my knee as intact as I could. So there I was, approaching the first mile marker and caught up with a group of other runners (me in my big knee brace) when one of the guys next to me told his running buddy, "Perfect pace. Just under six-thirty." I sort of freaked out a bit. While I may have felt comfortable in my mind, that was the fastest mile I had run since my injury, and by over 30 seconds. I had yet to break the 7:00-mile mark post-injury.

I took a few good breaths and reminded myself that I was committed no matter what happened over the course of the next 12 miles.

Just past the three-mile mark was the first spot that Jenny could cheer me on from. As I turned the corner and she came into view, I could see a shock-and-awe expression on her face. The only other thing I remember besides her cheering, is that I tossed her my Oakley's because the overcast wasn't burning off.

From then on, it was me and the other runners with a few spots of spectators and water stations along the route. The only time marker on the course was at the halfway point. I went through and immediately started calculating the average mile pace in my head. I was just under 7:00-mile pace for the first 6.55 miles, and people started passing me.

As I approached the 10-mile marker, my left leg went essentially numb, from the top of the brace down. By this point, I was getting consistently passed by other runners. It felt like I was going slower than my slowest jog, but nothing was going to stop me from finishing.

At about mile 12, a fellow runner with a distinctive hat (it was a visor with fake maroon colored spiky hair like a wig attached) took his hat off as he passed me and yelled out, "Hats off to you!" That was pretty motivational and timely, because I was struggling to keep going.

After I crossed the finish line, I saw my wife and kids. They were behind a fence that kept spectators out of the finish area. I tried to get over to them, but I kept walking in a small circle because I just couldn't get my left leg to work right any longer. I finally reached them, and it was one of the best moments of my life. Even though I was 60th overall and third in my age group, I felt happier than when I'd won state titles.

As I walked through the finisher's party area, I found myself next to the runner who took his hat off to me. He made it a point to shake my hand and asked about my injury. I briefly told him, and he was shocked that it was only five months previous. He then asked, "Why would you run this race and not defer the entry to next year?" I replied, "Because God told me to." That led to a brief conversation about God and following His voice.

I don't know if that man knew God before that conversation or not, but I'm certain that God had me run that race specifically for that conversation to happen.

God works that way sometimes. I could have easily not attempted that trick on water skis, or I could have fallen without being injured to that extreme. But it happened and God made a great thing happen because of it. Had I never suffered that knee injury, I probably could have placed in the top 10-20 runners that year and won my age group. It would have been no big deal to anyone but me and my family. We would have come home, and I'd have prepared for the next race.

Instead, God impacted someone's life through pushing me beyond what almost anyone else thought was possible. I don't know if anyone else was specifically impacted at that race that day by me being there, but one man was. I can only assume that God used that one connection to create a ripple effect upon the people that the runner interacted with afterwards.

That's what living a life with No More Sugar Coating is about. Not just being the person God has called you to be, but showing others that they can be the person they are called to be.

The late Kobe Bryant summed it up perfectly in his book, *The Mamba Mentality: How I Play*. He wrote:

> *"When I was young, my mindset was image, image, image. I took that approach with the media. As I became more experienced I realized: No matter what, people are going to like you or not like you. So be authentic, and let them like you or not for who you actually are."*

Once Bryant came to that realization, he was much more candid with reporters. He stopped giving them what they wanted to hear and simply gave short and sweet, truthful answers.

My mindset as a runner has changed. When I was younger, it was all about winning the race. While I still enjoy winning races, or at least winning my age group, I now run to show my core beliefs. I run for God. I run to hopefully inspire others to do something active for their own health. I run because it's a gift God gave me, and that is a part of who I am at the core. If I didn't run, I would be sugar coating who I am, in turn, denying the world around me.

In 2017, I started an annual effort of running to raise money for the Hewitt Public Library, which has transformed into the Running for Readers 5k event.

Why the library? I made a commitment on July 29, 2017, to reach a point where I was reading one book a week. Reading is what the most successful individuals in life do on a regular basis. I didn't hit that goal in 2017, 2018, or 2019 but read a total of 71 books over that time period. As of this writing in mid-2020, I'm slightly ahead of the one-book-a-week goal for this year. Not bad for a guy who got a D in fourth-grade reading and didn't read more than five books total in the 25 years since high school.

Through all these books, I've learned many great lessons. The biggest lesson is that you can find happiness through any number of ways—faith, family, sports, work—but you won't find true happiness until you break the sugar-coated layer of your life and give the world who you are.

The world needs you! We need you to be you! Sure, it's scary, and it's hard to stand out from the crowd. I challenge you to break free from the sugar coating, today.

You won't regret it!

Live who you are!

Go get your happiness!

# 14 Commitments to a Life Without Sugar-Coating

Commitment #1: Honesty - make a commitment to always be truthful

- Timeframe: Right Now
- Vision: What would life be like if everything you said was a truthful statement?

Commitment #2: Stop judging yourself

- Timeframe: Right Now
- Vision: Imagine your future self being happy with who you are

Commitment #3: Share an opinion derived from one of your core beliefs with a friend. Pick something which that friend doesn't already know about you.

- Timeframe: In the next 48 hours
- Vision: Sharing freely with friends when times are both great and difficult

Commitment #4: Volunteer at an organization that fits with you values

- Timeframe: In the next 7 days
- Vision: Make a long-term decision to volunteer on a regular basis

Commitment #5: Add a 5-minute pause to your morning routine. Sit quietly with no distractions, breath deeply, and repeat positive affirmations about who you are and what you offer the world (saying them out loud adds to the effectiveness)

- Timeframe: Daily, starting tomorrow morning
- Vision: See all the positive outcomes that are possible when you believe in yourself

Commitment #6: Try something new that is outside your comfort zone

- Timeframe: In the next 7 days
- Vision: See yourself as bold and courageous

Commitment #7: Schedule and complete a consumption inventory

- Timeframe: In the next 14 days
- Vision: A life where you recognize the negative inputs before they become a part of your life

Commitment #8: Identify something you believe simply because a "trusted source" told you. Research for yourself to determine if you truly believe it.

- Timeframe: In the next 14 days
- Vision: Constant learning provides wisdom that will be invaluable to future decision making

Commitment #9: Contact your 3-5 closest friends and ask them to hold you accountable to living free of sugar-coating

- Timeframe: In the next 7 days
- Vision: A future with strong friendships, lifting each other up, and celebrating great achievements together

Commitment #10: Make another attempt at something you failed at in the past

- Timeframe: In the next 7 days
- Vision: See yourself as someone who does not give up easily

Commitment #11: Write down 3 positive goals to achieve each day, check them off as they are completed

- Timeframe: Daily in the morning starting tomorrow
- Vision: See yourself smiling as you go to bed each night knowing you had a positive impact on the world that day

Commitment #12: Have faith in the plan God has for you

- Timeframe: Always
- Vision: Arriving in Heaven and hearing the words "Well done my good and faithful servant!"

Commitment #13: Read books about the subject matter of your life's purpose

- Timeframe: Daily
- Vision: Having the wisdom and courage to help your community grow and prosper

Commitment #14: Create a list of 3 things each day that you are grateful for

- Timeframe: Daily before bed for 21 days, starting today
- Vision: Living a life where you spend more time acknowledging the positives in your life instead of dwelling on the negatives

# Acknowledgements

First off, I have to thank my wife, Jenny for her constant, unwavering support. We've had some twists and turns in our 20+ years of marriage, but I would not have wanted to be on this ride with anyone else. Thank you for putting up with my unorthodox schedule as an entrepreneur, athlete, author, and coach. Just being next to you brings me more joy and peace than anything else in the world.

My children, Abigail and Tai, have possibly taught me more than I've taught them. It's amazing how much you can learn about life simply by parenting.

I can't thank Lynne Klippel and her team at Starmaker Communications enough. Lynne, you have once again guided me to the creation of a book I almost thought wouldn't happen. Over a year ago, I emailed you with an idea that, through time became this book. Thanks for always being there with advice (sometimes the tough advice to hear) and for being patient through the development process. Dustin Bilyk streamlined my thought process writing style into the clear and concise finished manuscript. Angie Grant captured my vision for the cover in a way I couldn't have imagined. Kaz Morran did a tremendous job editing and trying to make sense of my sometimes-illiterate writing. Lynne, you have a great team! You have all been a blessing to work with!

A special thank you to my church family that have been so supportive of my journey into entrepreneurship. Matt, Grant, James,

Josef, Tom, Ryan, Thomas, Pastor Grant, and so many others - you have prayed faithfully for my family in a way that I know glorifies God. I just hope my prayers for you and your families are as powerful.

I am particularly grateful to my athletes, clients, employees, and podcast listeners - thank you for allowing me to help you reach your goals. It's an honor to work with each of you. To my podcast guests, I have gained knowledge from each of you. Thank you for taking the time to teach both me and my listeners how to be healthier and better people.

I am eternally thankful for my high school coach, Pete Boudreaux. Now that I'm on the coaching side of the sports world, I find myself thanking God every day that you were my coach. Pete, I lean on your principles and example with every practice I lead. I would be nowhere near the coach I am without you.

I want to acknowledge Chris Rosser for accepting my request to disciple me. Many of our conversations are represented in this book.

Lastly, I would be remiss if I did not acknowledge the support that my friend Charles McCulloch has been to me. Whether in coaching, in business, or just as friends, you've been there to help me stay motivated, stay grounded, and keep living my core values even when we disagree.

# About the Author

Jerry Snider is an author, entrepreneur, podcast host, coach, and athlete. After growing up in Baton Rouge, he moved back to his birth state to attend Texas A&M University on a Track & Field scholarship. Earning a degree in exercise physiology, coupled with competing at a high level as a distance runner, has given Jerry the knowledge and tools to transform his client's health and wellness.

Jerry and his wife, Jenny, married in June of 2000 and have lived in Hewitt, Texas, since 2002. They have two children, Abigail and Tai. The Sniders are members of Fellowship Bible Church in Waco, Texas, where they have attended church since 2003. Jerry worked in various businesses and non-profits before opening his business, All In Health and Wellness, in 2016.

Jerry and Jenny purchased another business, Luna Juice Bar, in January 2020. Their hope is to continue to bring the message of health to the community through healthy meal options.

As a certified Life Breakthrough Coach, Jerry believes in a functional approach to solving problems. Discovering and eliminating the true source of pain (what is holding you back) is far more important than treating the symptoms. He has been cited in several articles, blog posts, and podcasts in regards to health, fitness, wellness, and entrepreneurship.

Volunteering in his community continues to be very important to Jerry. He served in Track & Field, Cross Country, and Football coaching roles with Texas Wind Athletics, helping the football team win the first ever Texas Homeschool State Football Championship in 2017. Jerry is in his third year as the Cross Country and Track Coach at Eagle Christian Academy in Waco, TX. Each year Jerry has coached, he has had at least one individual or relay state champion.

Jerry has been an active member of the City of Hewitt Parks and Beautification Board since 2018. He has volunteered in various ways at his church including as usher, speaker at retreats, LIFE group leader, and children's Sunday School leader. He also volunteers at multiple community events each year.

In October of 2017, Jerry developed a fundraiser for the City of Hewitt Public Library called All In with Jerry: Running for Readers. He raised $2,000 for the library to expand its selection of books for business owners. To generate awareness for the campaign, Jerry ran every foot of the 258 streets in Hewitt, covering 156 miles in 21 days. With the help of the Hewitt Library, the inaugural Running for Readers 5k occurred in January 2020. To date, Running for Readers has expanded the business section of the library by over 100 books.

Snider launched the Confidence Through Health podcast in 2019. Appropriately named after his first book, *Confidence Through Health*, the weekly episodes strive to provide insight into all areas of a healthy lifestyle.

You can contact Jerry at jerry@allinhealthandwellness.com with any questions or comments about health and wellness.

To find out more, go to www.allinhealthandwellness.com, and you can subscribe to the podcast at www.confidencethroughhealth.com or search for it on Apple Podcasts.

www.ingramcontent.com/pod-product-compliance
Lightning Source LLC
Chambersburg PA
CBHW070839300326
41935CB00038B/1148